PENG

IT WAS PROBABLY SOMETHING YOU ATE

Nicols Fox is a journalist whose work has appeared in *The Economist*, *The New York Times*, *The Washington Post*, *Lear's*, *Newsweek*, *The Boston Globe*, *USA Today*, *The Christian Science Monitor*, *American Journalism Review*, *Los Angeles Times*, *The Atlanta Journal-Constitution*, *Columbia Journalism Review*, *The Washingtonian*, *Art in America*, and many other publications. She has appeared on numerous radio and television programs as an expert on foodborne illness, including *48 Hours*, *Today*, and *Nightline* with the U.S. Secretary of Agriculture. She is the author of *Spoiled: Why Our Food Is Making Us Sick and What We Can Do about It*, also published by Penguin Books.

It Was Probably
SOMETHING
You ATE

A Practical Guide to Avoiding
and Surviving Foodborne Illness

Nicols Fox

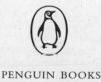

PENGUIN BOOKS

PENGUIN BOOKS
Published by the Penguin Group
Penguin Putnam Inc., 375 Hudson Street,
New York, New York 10014, U.S.A.
Penguin Books Ltd, 27 Wrights Lane, London W8 5TZ, England
Penguin Books Australia Ltd, Ringwood, Victoria, Australia
Penguin Books Canada Ltd, 10 Alcorn Avenue,
Toronto, Ontario, Canada M4V 3B2
Penguin Books (N.Z.) Ltd, 182–190 Wairau Road,
Auckland 10, New Zealand

Penguin Books Ltd, Registered Offices:
Harmondsworth, Middlesex, England

First published in Penguin Books 1999

1 3 5 7 9 10 8 6 4 2

A NOTE TO THE READER
The ideas, procedures, and suggestions contained in this book
are not intended as a substitute for medical treatment by a
physician. They reflect the author's experiences, studies, research,
and opinions. The information included in this publication is
believed to be accurate. Neither the author nor the publisher are
responsible for any adverse effects or consequences resulting from
the use of this material.

LIBRARY OF CONGRESS CATALOGING IN PUBLICATION DATA
Fox, Nichols.
It was probably something you ate: a practical guide to avoiding
and surviving foodborne illness/Nichols Fox.
p.   cm.
Includes bibliographical references.
ISBN 0 14 02.7799 4
1. Foodborne diseases—Popular works.   I. Title.
RC143.F69   1999
615.9´54—dc21   98–52910

Printed in the United States of America
Set in Bembo
DESIGNED BY BETTY LEW

Contents

Preface

There is nothing more important to people than a predictable and steady supply of safe food and water. All other desires pale in the face of this need. Yet there is a growing awareness that our assumptions about food safety have been optimistic if not entirely misplaced. Outbreaks of foodborne illness make the news with increasing frequency, drawing attention precisely because they are caused by more virulent pathogens, they are linked to foods previously thought to be safe, they are larger than outbreaks in the past, or they are caused by microbes that a few years ago no one had heard of. As all these things happen, there is a growing realization that what we once thought we knew about foodborne disease no longer applies. Old ideas about what is safe and what is not have had to be replaced. The rules for how foods must be handled in our kitchens, restaurants, and in processing plants have had to be rewritten. The complacent attitude consumers have about who is responsible for food safety needs revision.

My first book on this topic, *Spoiled*, told of the ecological causes of the constantly shifting pattern of foodborne disease. The conclusions of that book: We have changed everything about our relationship to food, and by opening windows to emerging foodborne pathogens, these changes are making us sick. It seemed obvious, given the response to *Spoiled*, that something more on the topic was needed: a focused, practical guide to avoiding and surviving these new foodborne threats.

Even as I was writing, the scene was changing. A pathogen that had been only rarely seen, *Vibrio parahaemolyticus,* caused illnesses in seven states after victims ate contaminated oysters. *Escherichia coli* O157:H7 made 26 children very ill and killed one after they swam in chlorinated water at a popular water park. *Salmonella agona,* usually found in the animal-protein component of animal feed, was discovered after more than a hundred related illnesses to have contaminated a toasted breakfast cereal, necessitating a wide-ranging recall. After sprouts were found to be the source of various pathogenic organisms in different outbreaks, the Food and Drug Administration (FDA) advised that anyone with an impaired immune system should avoid eating them. In Illinois 4,000 people were made sick by a strain of *E. coli* normally seen only in developing countries. Despite new food-safety regulations, outbreaks of *E. coli* O157:H7 and recalls of contaminated hamburger continued. As publication neared, an outbreak caused by *Listeria*, which resulted in 16 deaths and multiple recalls of hot dogs and lunchon meats, alerted the public to yet another hazard in familiar foods.

I am not a physician or a scientist. I am a journalist. In writing this book I have turned to the scientific and medical community, to the medical and scientific literature, to public documents, and to individuals who have been stricken by foodborne disease. The descriptions of their personal experiences were conveyed through interviews I conducted. The information about specific pathogens comes from a number of different sources including the Centers for Disease Control and Prevention (CDC), the U.S. Department of Agriculture, the FDA, the Council for Agricultural Science and Technology, and experts in the field. Where their information has differed—as in how long an illness is apt to last—I have adopted the widest range of opinion. When I supplement these references with my own personal opinion, it will be obvious. Where treatments are mentioned, that information comes from CDC documents as well but is meant as a reference only and not as a substitute for medical advice from your physician.

My purpose in writing this book is not to frighten. Eating can— and certainly should—still be a pleasure. But information is power, and my hope is that armed with the facts individuals can apply what they know, not only to keeping themselves and their families as safe as possible, but to making change.

I want to thank all those individuals who shared their experiences with me—and with the reader. These stories make the topic come alive, and I am grateful for their generosity. I also want to thank Dr. Kathleen Gensheimer, state epidemiologist of Maine, who has been unfailingly supportive and helpful for many years. I also want to thank my generous and attentive editor, Edward Iwanicki, who gave this project much time and care. Any errors are mine and mine alone.

1

Who Spoiled Food?

You can't define it, but you don't feel quite right. You're not interested in food, not interested in much of anything, really. You think you might have a bit of fever—your forehead seems damp—but you're not curious enough to take your temperature even if a thermometer were handy. You feel lethargic and vaguely out of sorts, quick to become irritated and to speak sharply. Once or twice your bowels rumble a warning. Then it hits; a sudden cramp grips your lower abdomen. You are hot and sweaty. Your body is clearly in trouble. The pain is sharp but bearable. Then it is gone and you feel cool again, perhaps too cool. Certainly not well. You keep on doing whatever you are doing—entertaining a client, discussing the new phone system with your boss, sitting in the dentist's chair, driving an 80,000-pound rig down the interstate, pontificating on a talk show, working on a deadline story, trying to impress a date—but your mind is busily making plans, because you fear what's coming. You may feel nausea—compelling nausea. Your intestines are in turmoil. Even without medical knowledge, you know you've been hit by something undesirable.

You might think of it as a "bug" or you may call it "the flu," which it is not. (Influenza is a respiratory disease.) Very likely, enemy bacteria have invaded your digestive system, multiplying until they have overwhelmed the ability of the usual microbial residents to compete with and conquer an unfriendly intruder. The enemies are now victorious and in control, creating havoc in an effort to have their way, perhaps producing toxins that may be damaging the very cells of your body. The invaders have a simple goal: to multiply in a friendly environment and survive by the millions, at your expense, then to move on. If the bacterial or viral load is heavy, it could mean days of incapacitation with both diarrhea and vomiting. The nausea might strike at an unfortunate moment, as it did the president of the United States on an official visit to Japan, when he threw up on an official's shoe at a formal gathering in full view of the world's television cameras.

If you recover on your own in a day or two, count yourself lucky. You've probably just had a mild episode, a self-resolving episode, of foodborne illness. It's happened to most of us, for some, many times over.

It could have been worse. It might have sent you to the hospital. It might have meant restoring fluids and salts intravenously, or surgery or intensive care to support organs damaged by the attack. In the most serious infections that develop into hemolytic uremic syndrome, for instance, you might have been left with a colostomy, reactive arthritis, a lifelong impairment of the digestive system, or damage to the lungs, the kidneys, the brain, or the heart. You might have been more seriously affected if you were immunocompromised in some way: at the extremes of age, undergoing chemotherapy, a transplant recipient, an AIDS patient, or even if you were simply taking antibiotics or had recently been ill. If you had been pregnant, the infection might have brought on a miscarriage or resulted in an infant with birth defects.

Or it might have killed you.

The infection could have come from something you ate or drank that morning, or a week ago or even longer, depending on the particular culprit. It might have been a raw food, a contaminated cooked food, an undercooked food, a dried food, or even a frozen food. It might have been a commercial food product, or something served at a restaurant, or a dish you you cooked yourself. You'll probably never know, and now that it's over, you probably don't care.

In an anything-goes era it's odd that we're still uncomfortable talking about an illness almost as common as the cold but potentially more serious. Diarrheal disease kills more people around the world than any other single illness, but the worst numbers come from countries where sanitation conditions are poor and where drinking water may be polluted. Until very recently we in developed countries have not appreciated how serious the illnesses can be where sanitation is good and water supplies are generally clean and safe. If television ads for diarrhea medication are an indication of how the public feels, diarrheal disease is a kind of bad joke. Recently, as outbreaks have increased, as some of the severe illnesses and deaths have become public and the press and consumers have paid more attention, it doesn't seem quite as funny anymore.

This is what the experts know: that diarrheal illness related to the foods we eat strikes millions and kills many thousands in the United States each year. Yet exactly how many cases there are is a matter of hot debate with political and economic consequences. An admission of too many cases would reflect badly on the federal agencies whose duty it is to safeguard food. Thus the relevant agencies have agreed among themselves to a number, a compromise among various estimates—33 million cases a year with 9,000 deaths, the food-safety and public health officials now say—but behind the united surface there is wide disagreement. When President Bill Clinton announced new safe-food regulations in 1996, making public this agreed-upon number, export orders for U.S. meats fell and meat producers complained. The numbers were far too high, they said, and were hurting their business. Yet studies by other credible scientists report even higher numbers, their estimates, based on careful calculations from community surveys, ranging from 81 million to 99 million Americans made ill each year. One expert at the Centers for Disease Control and Prevention in Atlanta thinks that each of us has at least one episode of foodborne disease a year, which would put the number at more than 260 million cases. Even the U.S. Department of Agriculture (USDA), conflicted as it is with the mandate to support U.S. agriculture even as it attempts to ensure safe food (thus with no incentive to exaggerate), puts the annual cost of foodborne illness in the United States at between $5.6 billion and $9.4 billion; a congressional committee report estimates it at $22 billion.

There is a great deal of pressure to come up with new numbers and the CDC was in the process of doing that as this book was being readied for publication. A source within the agency says that "the number of cases of foodborne diseases will be similar to previous estimates. The number of deaths are likely to decline but will still be remarkably high."

What the experts also know is that foodborne disease is woefully undercounted when it comes to officially reported cases. The reasons why are obvious. People usually treat themselves. If a victim does seek medical care, the illness may be misdiagnosed. A stool culture may not be taken. Even if a culture is made, or the stool examined for parasites, the lab may not find the responsible organism. Even if the culprit is identified, reporting to public health authorities is inconsistent and sometimes delayed. Rarely are fines administered for failure to report. Those who specialize in foodborne disease know that for every case reported, as many as 50 or 99 or even 199 may not be.

Foodborne disease is caused by bacteria, viruses, and parasites, most of them tiny creatures commonly referred to as microbes. The illnesses they produce, many of which have similar symptoms, are usually transmitted by what is known as the fecal-oral route. Somehow human or animal waste carrying the pathogens (the technical name for microbes that cause disease) is passed from person to person by hands or common objects. Or the pathogens transported in human and animal waste get onto the food we eat or into the water we drink.

Bacteria in hamburgers, parasites on raspberries, viruses in strawberries, outbreaks caused by microbes on salad greens and alfalfa sprouts—it seems hardly a week passes when Americans aren't confronted by more bad news about food. Old microbes appear in new foods—foods we once considered safe. Day after day we discover that foods we have eaten our entire lives have suddenly become dangerous. Chicken, turkey, eggs, staples of the diet—all are responsible for numerous illnesses. Autumn treats such as fresh apple cider, or age-old preservation techniques that create cured, dry salami, are suddenly called into question. Foodborne disease is clearly serious business, but is it really a new problem or are we just hearing about it more often?

Actually, both are happening. We have old microbes in new places, and we have familiar microbes that are now either more easily identified as the cause of human disease or present in greater numbers than ever before and thus more obviously causing illness. We also truly have new emerging disease-causing organisms, created through mutation or conjugation, infiltrating the food supply; pathogens unheard of twenty years ago have now spread around the globe. Some older microbes are showing new virulence or are developing strains resistant to antibiotics. It all spells serious trouble.

Clean, safe food is so fundamental to our sense of well-being that contaminated food begins to feel like betrayal. Because we have such a resistance to thinking that what is essential to our health and nourishment might make us sick or kill us, some of us take refuge in denial. We don't want to know. Yet to be unaware of the risks and how they can be avoided is to be especially vulnerable. It is also equally dangerous to assume that our past experience is relevant to the situation today. "I've eaten sunny-side eggs all my life and they've never hurt me," says an older friend, not realizing that eggs have changed just in the last decade. What was safe a generation ago, whether a raw oyster or a pink hamburger, is not necessarily a risk-free option today.

As federal agencies and the food industry attempt to shift responsibility to the consumer with the oft-heard "if only they would just cook it" mantra, the consumer is suddenly plunged into a brave new world where food preparation is a treacherous undertaking. Cooks are expected to become virtual lab technicians in biohazard environments, scrubbing down before and after preparing foods, disinfecting, avoiding cross-contamination, sterilizing. The bewildered consumer can be forgiven for recoiling with surprise and asking, "What happened to food?"

Foodborne disease has changed because we have changed. Everything about the way we raise food animals and crops, as well as the way we slaughter, process, transport, distribute, and sell foods, has been transformed in the past 50 years. As consumers we no longer buy and prepare foods the way we once did. Today our priorities are convenience, novelty, year-round availability, and low cost. The formal family dinner as a command performance is virtually a thing of the past. We eat out more often, content to leave food preparation and safety to some of our lowest paid workers without questioning that irony. Increasingly we favor fresh fruits and vegetables for health reasons without considering that raw foods, especially those that first travel the globe, then go through hands-on processing, present their own particular risks.

Packaging and advertising coupled with confidence in federal regulation—that feeling that someone out there is protecting us—have lulled consumers into a sense of complacency about food safety. These new expectations, combined with the other changes, are opening doors to emerging foodborne pathogens.

We live in a microbial world. Microbes live by the billions on us and in us. They live around us, in the environment, and on and in the food animals and plants that we consume. Most are benign and some are actually helpful. Some are essential to digestion and the absorption of nutrients in our guts. Any change at all in the environment, including the smallest changes in how we do something—prepare a dish, for instance—has the potential to open the door to an opportunistic and aggressive microbe on the lookout for a more favorable spot to settle down and raise a family. Alter the food a cow eats and the microbial equilibrium in the animal's gut is changed. The new atmosphere can invite in a new microbe. It was just such an innocent shift that now seems to have opened the door to the acid-resistant *Escherichia coli* O157:H7, one of the most vicious newcomers. At every step in the food chain from farm to fork, similar shifts have inadvertently invited in unfriendly intruders.

Once it was possible for federal officials and food producers to say with a straight face, "We have the safest food in the world." Today we have the world's food, and it is as safe as the environment from which it comes. The international food trade is equally as efficient at distributing pathogenic organisms as it is exotic delights. A woman in Baltimore becomes ill with cholera from imported frozen coconut juice from Thailand. Contaminated canned mushrooms from China cause illnesses across the country from *Staphylococcus aureus*. Imported shrimp in New Mexico cause a case of cholera. More and more frequently we are seeing these international interlopers infiltrating the products of the mindless global food exchange.

We know when we travel to developing countries to eat with care, but many of the foods in our produce counters are coming from these same countries, and we scarcely give a thought to whether they might be contaminated. In a local grocery store in

Maine the fruits and vegetables come from 26 different nations. When we consume this produce we forget that we are, in essence, consuming the soil and water in which they were grown and even the working, living, and sanitation conditions of those who picked and packed the products. Whether these harvesters have access to bathroom and hand-washing facilities can suddenly become very important when we eat the produce without further cooking. For two years in a row Guatemalan raspberries brought with them the unusual parasite *Cyclospora,* causing thousands of serious gastrointestinal infections. Imported cantaloupe, tomatoes, green onions, alfalfa sprouts, and strawberries have all been associated with outbreaks of foodborne disease. Sometimes even cooking isn't enough. In November 1996 five individuals who dined at a Montreal restaurant became ill with a rare toxin poisoning from eating barracuda imported from the Caribbean. Physicians now need to be prepared to deal with diseases and illnesses they've likely never heard of in a world where last night's dinner may have come from half a world away.

Foodborne disease is nothing new, but in the last 30 or 40 years it has changed in nature, numbers, and the pattern of infection. Once food outbreaks were local—the spoiled potato salad at the family reunion was a typical example. These were outbreaks easy to spot because nearly everyone got sick—except cousin Lucy who never ate potato salad, which neatly pointed to the cause. Often blame could be placed on an infected food handler, a prepared food that had been left out at room temperature, and the bacterium *Staphylococcus aureus.*

Now the picture has changed. Not entirely, of course. The small local outbreaks still occur. But today outbreaks may be national or even international in scope as contaminated mass-produced and widely distributed foods embark on their cosmopolitan travels. As outbreak follows outbreak the public is learning a string of tongue-twisting names—the new culprits in foodborne disease: *E. coli* O157:H7, *Campylobacter, Listeria, Yersinia, Cryptosporidium,* hepatitis A, *Cyclospora, Salmonella enteritidis.* You can't, as in the past, look to your last meal as the cause of illness, since some of these new bugs may take longer to wreak gastrointestinal havoc. This makes incriminating the food that carried the infection difficult or unlikely. And mass distribution may well mean that cases don't occur in groups but are scattered all across the country in what seem, at first, to be sporadic, random infections. In 1994 mass-produced ice cream contaminated with *Salmonella* was identified as the culprit in an outbreak eventually estimated to have caused 224,000 illnesses in 48 states. It had an equal chance of going entirely undetected because of the spotty, random nature of mass-produced infection.

We've also changed how we manufacture foods. Often shifts in processes are made for what seem to be good reasons without considering whether or not the change will create a niche for a human pathogen. When a yogurt manufacturer in the United Kingdom replaced the sugar in hazelnut yogurt with artificial sweetener, that small alteration created a friendly medium for *Clostridium botulinum*. The result: 27 cases of botulism, a potentially fatal disease.

We've changed how we cook. Vegetables may be sold already washed and trimmed and cut to size, but by whom? Where? In what kind of water? Microwave ovens don't cook evenly and have been implicated in foodborne disease outbreaks where meat dishes have not been cooked or reheated sufficiently to kill bacteria. We like the ease of packaged salads, but in the "modified atmospheric packaging" in which many are sold—an environment that inhibits bacteria that simply cause spoiling but aren't disease-causing in humans—the more harmful pathogens that favor low-oxygen conditions may flourish.

Or we don't cook at all, preferring to buy plastic containers of prepared food. In the summer of 1997 the bacterium *Listeria monocytogenes,* which can cause a serious illness that in pregnant women can lead to miscarriage, was found in hummus sold nationwide. Because of poor manufacturing practices the Food and Drug Administration (FDA) was concerned about many of the company's products, which included tabbouleh, baba gannouj, salsa and other dips, and salads. The FDA asked for an immediate recall but later found, after checking, that products were still on supermarket shelves and retail store managers had never been informed of the danger. Another widespread recall from *Listeria*-contaminated food occurred in November 1997. In fact, a peek at the FDA recall lists reveals many, many recalls for *Listeria* that the public never hears about—recalls that are buried on the back pages of newspapers if they are printed at all. Did these products cause illness? Without testing and reporting, it was impossible to say. How many illnesses were passed off incorrectly as "the flu"? *Listeria monocytogenes* is a pathogen especially dangerous to pregnant women, yet where are the public warnings that they should avoid eating deli foods? How many miscarriages are actually related to infection with the bacteria?

As if to underscore that nothing is safe, even chocolate contaminated with *Salmonella* has caused illnesses in England, Scandinavia, Canada, and the United States. Contaminated heroin and marijuana have caused outbreaks from foodborne pathogens as well.

The global distribution of foodborne pathogens is a two-way street. We don't just import pathogens: we export them. In October 1997, Korean officials inspecting beef imports from the United States found *E. coli* O157:H7. Japan had found the bacteria on beef intestines from the United States two years earlier. But their own huge outbreak was linked to sprouts grown downstream from a cattle-raising area.

Travel and sophistication have expanded the eating horizons of middle-income Americans, and often we prepare foods we have little traditional experience with. Professionally trained sushi preparers know that raw fish can harbor parasitic worms and that ingesting one may result in emergency surgery, but how many of those who prepare sushi at home know to look for these worms? Or know to freeze the fish first (with the exception of salmon), a process which, if done properly, kills the worms.

Eating raw shellfish is a cultural tradition of long standing, but how many people know that as pollution levels rise in our coastal waters it is now considered to be highly risky? In one study, of those who eventually died from a pathogen called *Vibrio vulnificus,* 88 percent reported consuming raw oysters. Individuals with certain liver conditions are especially vulnerable.

We expect food to be cheap, consider it in the United States as almost a birthright, and yet constant pressure from consumers to keep food prices almost absurdly low has meant changes in how food is produced, processed, and distributed. Chicken was once reserved for Sunday dinner; now it is everyday fare and a quarter the price per pound of a yellow pepper. Why is it a surprise that the factory-farming methods that make chicken that cheap have also made it more likely to carry disease-causing bacteria? Subjecting intensively raised, virtually genetically identical animals to stresses such as overcrowding, antibiotics, contaminated feed, rough handling, and difficult conditions in transport makes these animals more susceptible to getting infections and passing them on to us. Some cattle are eating recycled chicken litter, saving money for cattle growers but an unsavory practice if ever there was one. Until very recently "rendered animal protein," composed of recycled dead and diseased animal parts, euthanized shelter animals, and other bits of meat considered unfit for human consumption, was being fed to dairy cattle, natural herbivores. It is still being fed to swine and poultry. This practice is assumed to be responsible for spreading "mad cow" disease in British beef and dairy herds. The FDA has now called a halt to feeding "ruminants to ruminants," as cud-chewing animals are called, but the practice continues to spread pathogens among poultry and some consumer advocates and industry critics doubt whether renderers will bother keeping the feed ingredients for the swine and poultry separate from the dairy cattle's feed, or whether federal regulators will have the resources or the will to enforce the regulation.

Vastly speeded-up modern slaughter can make contamination of raw animal products worse. Rubber plucking devices for chickens, conveyor belts in slaughterhouses, and water chill baths for poultry can—and do—spread bacteria from one carcass to another.

Even refrigeration, which has extended shelf life and improved food safety, has opened the door to pathogens, such as *Yersinia* and *Listeria,* that actually thrive in these chilly conditions. If processed products carry these bugs—and some are known to lurk in the processing environment—they can reproduce to dangerous levels during their long refrigerated shelf life.

Every step forward in food safety, every technological "improvement," seems to create a niche for a pathogen as microbes adapt and take advantage of situations that favor their comfort and well-being. Recommended cooking temperatures for killing pathogens in hamburger have risen in the last decade from 122°F to 165°F, leading some scientists to question whether we are in the process of creating heat-resistant bugs.

While raw animal products have always had the potential to carry pathogenic organisms, there is no doubt that eggs, poultry, and mass-produced hamburger are more contaminated today than ever before, and the finger points directly toward the intensive rearing of food animals and the mass processing and distribution of foods. When thousands of cows from up to four different countries meet at the mass grinders that now produce our hamburger and one contaminated cow can taint 16 tons of hamburger, expect trouble. That explains the massive recall in August 1997 of 25 million pounds of hamburger processed by Hudson Foods. When one discovers what actually goes into hamburger—the spent dairy cattle that no longer produce enough milk; the 25 percent cheek meat scraped from cattle heads; the 5 percent of "meat" from advanced meat recovery systems that use a high-pressure vacuum process to suck scraps from the spinal column, sometimes getting parts of spinal cord; the blood from the bottoms of the meat carts—it doesn't seem very appetizing at all, and the potential for it to be contaminated is hardly surprising. Dr. David Acheson of Tufts University in Boston sampled ground beef at his local supermarkets, looking not for *E. coli* O157:H7, which is difficult to find, but for the toxin it and other dangerous *E. coli* produce. He found it in 25 percent of the samples and confirmed the finding with further tests for the microbes.

Numbers aside, what is the threat of foodborne illness to ordinary people? There are tragic and dramatic stories of foodborne disease that are emotionally wrenching: a child who eats a hamburger and dies a week later after a hideous and excruciatingly painful illness; a woman left crippled for months after an infection with *Campylobacter;* an otherwise healthy young adult experiencing a long and debilitating illness following infection from *Cyclospora* in fresh-basil preparations; and a grown man who spends 12 days in intensive care, has three holes in his colon, and requires a colostomy after a bout of *Salmonella.* While most occurrences, in fact, are thankfully less serious, these severe cases happen often enough to demonstrate that none of us is exempt. Ordinary people doing ordinary things can have their lives altered or even ended by the simple act of taking a bite of an unsafe food. But a more typical and much less dramatic example of how foodborne disease can strike a family is the story told by Kay Harkins.

Kay's husband is a lieutenant colonel in the Marine Corps, stationed in Estonia. Kay stayed behind in their home in San Diego, California, where she teaches writing at Point Loma Nazarene College. She has two grown children, a 26-year-old daughter and a 22-year-old son. Her own encounter with foodborne disease followed an airline trip on which she was served a turkey sandwich. By the time she reached home she was feeling ill, and she was so sick by the next evening that "I thought I was going to die," she remembers.

There was no investigation to positively link Kay's turkey sandwich to her illness, but outbreaks from airline food are not that unusual. In 1988 a large proportion of the Minnesota Vikings football team began getting sick: the cases were eventually traced to sandwiches served by an airline. After an investigation it was estimated that 1,900 cases of infection with *Shigella* occurred after infected food handlers probably contaminated sandwiches they were preparing, which then weren't properly refrigerated before they were served. That outbreak was caught because of the football players. Illness in a group of high-profile individuals such as sports figures won't go unnoticed. There may well have been an outbreak connected to Kay's experience, but with travelers going in all directions the illnesses they experienced might not have been as clearly associated with what they ate on the plane. Many—in fact most—outbreaks of this nature probably escape identification.

Kay recovered in a week or so without medical help, but she's never felt quite the same about a turkey sandwich, guilty or not. And likewise many of us are losing our appetites as we hear about new outbreaks from everyday foods.

Kay's daughter fell victim to foodborne disease as well. She and her boyfriend ride mountain bikes, sometimes in Mexico. She thinks that's where she picked up a parasite called *Giardia lamblia*. Following one trip, she began having frequent bouts of diarrhea and nausea that simply wouldn't go away.

"She was always feeling on the verge of being sick," remembers Kay. Finally she was diagnosed and received treatment for the insidious and persistent bug.

In fact, *Giardia* is found in the United States, even in treated water supplies, as chlorination doesn't effectively kill it. It is present in water sources that are exposed to animal waste, such as reservoirs, and in tantalyzingly cool mountain streams where hikers sometimes drink. It is now a common cause of diarrheal disease in the United States. A public health official in New Mexico said it was the most frequent cause of failure to thrive in children in her area.

Kay got yet another lesson in foodborne disease when her daughter's boyfriend also developed serious stomach problems. His problems were eventually traced to infection with *Helicobacter pylori,* the bacteria now known to be responsible for about 80 percent of stomach ulcers. He could have contracted the infection from contaminated food or person-to-person contact—scientists are just learning how the infection is transmitted. Fortunately, a course of an antibiotic and drug combination can usually take care of the infection.

None of these illnesses was life threatening, but all were extremely unpleasant, debilitating, and an economic drain. Even uncultured, unidentified, and unreported foodborne disease takes its toll, both on individual well-being and on the community pocketbook through lost wages and other costs. Diarrheal disease is the stealthy hand in the pocket of our economy.

Kay Harkins is not only more conscious of what she eats now, she is more alert to the obvious violations of food safety that many of us are exposed to every day. Just one bad experience has damaged the trust she had in the safety of what she eats, and she is not alone. Once the breach was made, the carefully constructed message that our food is safe began crumbling almost as quickly as did the Berlin Wall.

We are entering into a new era of consciousness about food. The pathogens it can carry and their potential to make us sick or to kill us is coming as a shock to many Americans. In the era of modern medicine, we had, it seems, almost forgotten about germs, the popular word for microbes. They were once everywhere. And they caused disease. But with the discovery and rapid spread in the use of antibiotics, infectious diseases became less important, and worrying about "germs" had an old-fashioned ring to it. Expectations for personal cleanliness have become so standard—The Saturday-night bath or twice-a-year hair-washing of great-grandmother's day sounds appalling now—that we seemed to forget why cleanliness was once such a focus of attention. In the minds of teachers and parents, hand washing took a backseat to worries about drugs, violence, and teen pregnancy.

Yet not only have the "germs" stayed with us, they are more plentiful than ever on some of the foods we eat. At the same time, our most potent weapons of choice against the subsequent infections pathogenic microbes may cause have become less effective as antibiotic resistance grows. (Antibiotics are, in fact, seldom needed to treat foodborne disease, but when infections run amok, they become desperately important.)

Over the last few decades we have become remarkably complacent as well about the potential for food to make us ill. There are several reasons for the change. Advances in food technology and in packaging are reassuring. Refrigeration gives a false confidence that microbes can't develop or invade that sacred space, when in fact refrigerators are full of microbes that are merely slowed—not stopped. (Witness the growth on the tomato sauce you forgot in the far reaches of the bottom shelf.) Federal meat inspection, which began in 1907 following Upton Sinclair's revealing novel about the meat industry, *The Jungle*, has been assumed to be diligent and exacting. Yet *E. coli* O157:H7 is the only one of all the pathogenic organisms whose discovery on a raw food product can trigger a request to a company to recall the product. Raw animal foods contaminated with other pathogenic organisms still meet USDA standards. (Cooked, ready-to-eat foods have different standards.)

Industry, the USDA, and the FDA have all played a role in assuring Americans that they are buying safe food. In the past the customer questioned the sellers of food; now we have become conditioned and content to leave food safety to others, reassured that someone is keeping a close watch. Yet while some foods are safer, others have become more contaminated.

The methods used for rearing, slaughtering, and processing poultry today, though successful in bringing down the price, have also virtually guaranteed that chicken is contaminated with one pathogen or another. The USDA's own baseline studies found that "more than 99 percent" of poultry sampled was positive for generic *E. coli,* which is an indication that it has been contaminated with fecal material and thus has the potential to carry pathogens. Experts say "virtually all" chickens are contaminated with *Campylobacter,* an organism most Americans have not heard of but which, in fact, causes more foodborne illness than any other single pathogen and can lead to chronic diseases. There is a close connection between the use of antibiotics in chicken rearing—which makes chickens grow faster and prevents disease—and the presence of *Campylobacter.* The careless use of antibiotics in animal husbandry is now producing resistant strains of microbes that are infecting humans, so that some antibiotics are becoming useless in treating the illnesses in humans these pathogens produce.

Just a decade or two ago *Salmonella enteritidis* was rare inside eggs. Now it is a problem all across the United States and indeed around the world. The industry, and even public health officials, tend to blame the cook for undercooking the eggs, and yet hundreds of years of traditional cooking practices and thousands of familiar recipes that included undercooked eggs did not make people sick—until recently. The finger of blame can be pointed directly at the intensive approach to egg production: the limited diversity in the laying flocks, contaminated feed and water, and the crowding and stressing endured by the birds. The overuse of antibiotics is also linked to the problem. In June 1998 the USDA admitted that eggs were causing nearly 900,000 illnesses in the United States each year—a number they quickly retracted and revised to 650,000 cases—still far too many. Even at that rate, contaminated eggs are killing an estimated 650 people a year, based on the standard death rates for *Salmonella.*

Blame for the increase in foodborne disease can be placed squarely on an industry focused on spending less to earn more; on news media that only now are beginning to pay attention to a developing problem and the facts behind the increase in foodborne disease; on a government agency mired in conflict and far too cozy with the industry it is meant to regulate; on a political process and politicians all too dependent on money from agriculture-industry lobbyists; on a public health system that is often unable to identify the common source of random illnesses produced by mass-produced and widely distributed foods; and finally, on consumer demands for novelty, year-round availability, convenience, and, perhaps most critically, cheap food.

"Cheap is not cheap," a Chinese expression goes. Saving a dollar or two on chicken that results in an infection with *Salmonella* or *Campylobacter* is no savings at all. Yet our Agriculture Department has had, for several generations, a cheap-food policy. It's time that changed too, because it's making us sick. In the meantime, it's important to meet the enemy; to know what we're up against in the effort to eat safely. The following pages describe the organisms responsible for foodborne disease, how they cause illness, where they are likely to be found, and how to avoid them.

2

The Pathogens

THE BASIC SCIENCE

The thriving world of the tiny creatures that live on us, in us, and all around us was only revealed in 1674 or thereabouts by Antonie van Leeuwenhoek (1632–1723), a merchant, an amateur scientist, and clearly a man with an obsession—not for the creatures, which he knew nothing about, but for lenses. By carefully grinding a glass disk, he could see things larger than they actually were. While peering at a drop of water one day through a lens that he had ground, he saw amazing activity—tiny beasts, he called them, that swam about, playing almost. In a sense, that sight changed the world—or at the very least, enlarged it immensely. Leeuwenhoek went on to find the creatures virtually everywhere he looked. He also discovered that excessive heat could kill them—an important observation.

Because of the work of scientists who followed, such as Francesco Redi (1626–97) and Lazzaro Spallanzani (1729–99), microbes were soon revealed not to arise spontaneously, as has been thought, but to reproduce by division. Louis Pasteur (1827–95) and John Tyndall (1820–93) took the understanding of microorganisms further. Pasteur revealed that microbes have both useful and dangerous roles in human activity; he was one of the first to link the tiny creatures and disease. He was also the first to divide bacteria into those that required oxygen to grow (aerobic) and those that couldn't grow in its presence (anaerobic). Today it is well known that certain kinds of bacteria can grow and thrive under extreme conditions of heat and cold that other creatures find intolerable.

Credit for the specific linking of a particular organism to a particular disease goes to Agostino Bassi (1773–1856), who traced a disease in silkworms to a fungal infection; the work was confirmed by Pasteur. Joseph Lister (1827–1912), an English physician, is credited with using the growing understanding of microbes and their link to infection to devise antiseptic techniques for avoiding postoperative infection.

The late nineteenth century saw a rush of scientific activity that would uncover the microbes responsible for a number of serious illnesses. Robert Koch (1843–1910) applied a disciplined approach to medical microbiology. To confirm that a particular microbe did cause a specific illness demanded a step-by-step process. Still used today, the steps he devised are called Koch's postulates. Before an organism can be said to cause an illness, the following are required: (1) The same organism must be found in all cases of a given disease. (2) The organism must be isolated and grown in pure culture. (3) The organisms from the pure culture must reproduce the disease when inoculated into a susceptible animal. (4) The organism must then again be isolated from the experimentally infected animal. Koch, using his method, found the causes of anthrax, cholera, and tuberculosis.

The history of microbiology is filled with determined investigators who were humiliated and reviled for their claims about microorganisms and their means of transmission. Others caught or infected themselves with the illnesses they were investigating. Some died attempting to further our knowledge of disease.

To understand how microorganisms can cause foodborne disease, it is important to know something about them. Cells, of which all living organisms are formed, are of two types: prokaryotic and eukaryotic. Eukaryotic cells have intracellular membranes that compartmentalize the cell, making the structure more complex; they take 19 to 24 hours to divide. Fungi, molds, and yeast, as well as protozoa, those larger, filterable critters, such as *Cryptosporidium*, that cause waterborne diseases, are all eukaryotes.

Bacteria and cyanobacteria (blue-green algae) fall into the prokaryotic camp. Much simpler in organization, they divide quickly. One organism can become two in as little as 15 or 20 minutes, which for our purposes explains why foods should not be left to cool overnight on the kitchen counter.

That other category of troublemakers, viruses, are far tinier still and hover in that nebulous classification between living and not living. They actually exist and reproduce within host cells as parasites, and generally a cell infected with one dies. Viruses are not affected by antibiotics.

Bacteria cause most of the foodborne disease outbreaks. They are named according to the same system of classification devised for plants by Carolus Linnaeus in 1735. The bacteria within a given genus will have similar characteristics. *Salmonella* is a genus, and *typhi* a species, for example. There can be further divisions within a species and particular strains, or serotypes, of bacteria can be recognized by the characteristics of their DNA. It is possible today to link random cases of infection with *E. coli* O157:H7, for instance, by determining that the microbes responsible belong to the same genetic substrain.

Microbiologists can tell bacteria apart superficially under a microscope by looking at their shapes and sizes, whether they move about and how they do so (some have flagella, or whiplike structures, that they use to propel themselves), and additionally, how they accept stains, and how they live together in a colony. Further identification depends on different chemical characteristics, such as which sugars are metabolized, whether the organism can break down a certain substance, or on what media it will or will not grow.

Different terms are used to describe the appearance of bacteria. Some (cocci) look like tiny spheres or round berries under a microscope. Others have spiral forms (spirilla or spirochetes) or rod-shaped or cylindrical forms (called bacilli). While the flagella are long stringlike projections, bacteria may also have pili or fimbriae, which are small, hairlike structures that have different functions. Some bacteria form capsules made up of a secreted material that covers and can protect them under adverse conditions. They might ride out especially dry or hot times, for instance, until things get better.

Bacteria are often divided into gram-positive and gram-negative classifications, which is based on how the organism reacts to the Gram stain. The designation tells something about their cell walls.

Bacteria, like other organisms, need a constant supply of food to thrive and reproduce. They do well under certain temperature conditions and do poorly when out of their preferred range; they seldom thrive either in a very alkaline or a very acidic environment, although some species or even serotypes may be more tolerant of one or the other; and finally, some require oxygen and some do not. For some anaerobes, oxygen even has a lethal effect.

All this information is important for food safety because the objective is to keep bacteria that are harmful to humans from growing and reproducing in foods humans will consume. All food-safety techniques are directed toward that goal. To keep foods safe, one should know precisely those conditions that bacteria do not like (such as excessive acidity) or what can kill them (cooking) or keep them from growing (lack of oxygen for some or refrigeration for others). It's also important to realize that what kills one bacterium, such as a lack of oxygen, may be ideal for the growth of another. Or that while a certain amount of heat or acid is enough to kill one bacterium, it may not be enough to kill another.

Bacteria infect and cause illness in humans in different ways. *Staphylococcus aureus* used to be the favorite culprit in foodborne disease outbreaks. It has been replaced today by *Salmonella, Campylobacter,* and *Shigella,* but it is still around. It causes illnesses by producing a toxin that is released into food as it grows. Other pathogens may produce a toxin within the human body but take longer to cause an illness. *Bacillus cereus,* often found on rice, can actually cause two different kinds of illness, caused by the production of two different kinds of toxin. Some bacteria, such as *Shigella,* must first invade the epithelial cells of the intestine, where they secrete a toxin that eventually kills the cell. The ability to invade these intestinal cells is encoded in a plasmid within the cell. A plasmid is a bit of DNA within a bacterium that can replicate itself and can move from one bacterium to another through a method of reproduction called conjugation.

Drugs that can kill microorganisms are called antimicrobials or, more popularly, antibiotics. Bacteria may become resistant because (1) they can actually destroy the antibiotic, (2) a mutated form of the bacteria can become impermeable to the antibiotic, or (3) a mutated form has appeared that can resist the lethal effects of the antibiotics. Resistance to antibiotics can be transmitted from one cell to another by conjugation—call it the sex life of microbes—when plasmids are exchanged. The plasmid can also be transferred to different species of bacteria. Thus a plasmid within a *Salmonella* bacterium that makes it resistant to several different kinds of antibiotics can be transferred within a host organism, such as a human, to bacteria with the appropriate receptor sites, such as *Shigella* or *E. coli,* until they are all resistant to the antibiotics.

Now think for a moment about all of the characteristics just mentioned. Bacteria can reproduce quickly; they are adaptable, and there are species that can live virtually under any conditions; they can transfer traits, such as the ability to penetrate epithelial cells or to produce vicious toxins, among themselves; and they can develop and share resistance to antibiotics. Many of the organisms that cause human diseases have pretty efficient means of getting from one place to another via animal and human waste or water. Contemplating all of their advantages in a war between "us" and "them," we may find it hard to see the advantages we have. Probably the most important one is that we humans and other animals play a role in the life cycle of bacteria. Many grow well on us or in us, and many get from here to there in our waste. So lucky for us, they need us, and it's not in their interest to kill us off completely.

We cannot get along without microbes. To get along *with* them, it is important to understand their many and various characteristics, needs, and vulnerabilities. The sensible approach is to maintain an equilibrium or balance with the microbial world, realizing that wiping them out is not a possibility, nor would it be advisable. But learning to live with them in harmony just might be.

When a new foodborne disease appears or an outbreak occurs, Dr. Robert V. Tauxe at the Centers for Disease Control and Prevention says that in looking for the cause one should first ask, "What has changed?" Often some shift in human activity has opened the door, quite by accident, to a new microbe.

Whenever we close the door to one microbe, we open the door to another, and when dealing with food we'd better not forget that.

THE MAJOR PLAYERS

CAMPYLOBACTER JEJUNI

Alice Clair manages a gift shop in Bar Harbor, Maine. It's been a decade now since her encounter with *Campylobacter*, and she has to push her memory hard to recall some of the details as to precisely what happened and when. But she has no trouble at all remembering the pain and discomfort of the experience. Quite the contrary, she doubts the memory will ever go away.

It was in the summer of 1989 when Clair got together with friends one evening in Bangor, Maine. Barbecued chicken was on the menu at the backyard gathering, and she had her share. Not long afterward—a day or so, she thinks now—she began suffering cramps and then diarrhea and vomiting. Her illness was severe enough to put her in bed for several days. The diarrhea soon became bloody, and as in so many cases, that was enough to send her to the hospital emergency room.

"I was so sick," she says now, wincing at the memory.

It was fortunate she went. She was dehydrated, a condition that can have serious consequences. She was kept there for a few hours while she was rehydrated intravenously, and then she was sent home. The hospital took stool cultures and soon concluded that *Salmonella*, which they had suspected, *wasn't* the cause of her illness—at least the lab couldn't find the bacteria. The samples were submitted to further testing and something *was* found: a bacterium called *Campylobacter jejuni*.

The name meant nothing to Clair. It's a curious fact that the pathogen responsible for more foodborne disease than any other single organism is so unfamiliar to the general public. It only infrequently makes the news, perhaps for the simple reason that it is not easy to spell or pronounce (cám-pa-lo-bac-ter). But it is not an unfamiliar microbe to poultry producers. It doesn't cause poultry any problems, but it prefers the birds as a host. Today it is found on most of the raw poultry sold in the United States, where it is a potential source of illness to anyone who handles meat carelessly or fails to cook it thoroughly.

Clair was given an antibiotic to which the bacterium was susceptible, although it is not the generally recommended treatment. She gradually recovered, but she remembers that it wasn't overnight. In fact, it was weeks before she felt better, and even now she continues to have trouble with her bowels, which seems to be a common complaint among people who have had serious enteric infections.

Clair never knew for sure if the *Campylobacter* came from the barbecued chicken—no one else at the party became ill—but it easily could have, given its ubiquitous presence on poultry and the ease with which microbes of this sort can be transmitted, thereby cross-contaminating other foods. What might well have happened is that the chicken was seriously undercooked, or the barbecue sauce, applied throughout the cooking process with a brush, may have become contaminated from the initial contact with the raw poultry. Alice's piece of chicken might simply have been the one that received a swipe of contaminated sauce late in the cooking process, and the bacteria somehow avoided the heat and survived. One of the first documented outbreaks from *Campylobacter,* in 1982 in Colorado, was linked to barbecued chicken.

How this common pathogen could have eluded scientists as a cause of foodborne disease for so long is a tale worth telling. It doesn't mean that the bacterium wasn't around; it simply means that the connection had not yet been made between the illness and infection with the microbe. In fact, *Campylobacter*'s link to human disease became widely recognized only in 1977 when the *British Medical Journal* published an article by a British scientist, Martin Skirrow, entitled "*Campylobacter* Enteritis: A 'New' Disease." It would still be several years before the connection to food was solidly confirmed.

Campylobacter jejuni, the full name of the strain most likely to cause disease in humans, is a rod-shaped, gram-negative bacterium. It is slender, curved, and under a phase-contrast or a dark-field microscope the organisms can be seen to move around freely and gracefully, propelled by the flagella at each end. These tiny creatures have decided preferences for a warm, low-oxygen environment. The story of *Campylobacter*'s belated detection reveals a lot about science, research priorities, and the unfortunate division between human and animal medicine (now being somewhat corrected). *Campylobacter fetus* was originally called *Vibrio fetus* and was discovered as early as 1913 when its presence was linked to cattle and sheep that had aborted or were infertile. In the 1950s a researcher at the Centers for Disease Control and Prevention (CDC), the late Elizabeth King, felt that the organisms were more common than anyone realized but difficult to isolate. She did notice, however, that they were often found in the blood of people who reported having had diarrhea and that they were identical to those that veterinarians reported finding in chickens. In the early 1970s a Belgian physician, Jean-Paul Butzler, isolated the organism from a nurse in his lab and then claimed in the *Journal of Pediatrics* and the *Journal of Infectious Diseases* to have found it in 5 percent of children with diarrhea in a Moroccan community in Brussels—a startling proposal.

In England Martin Skirrow read the articles and was fascinated, but skeptical. Nevertheless, he followed up using Butzler's technique of isolating the organism using filtration and a culture medium that contained antibiotics. He at once got positives. It seems that *Campylobacter* is "fastidious," or hard to find, and easily overwhelmed in an ordinary culture by more aggressive microbes. These competitors were killed off by using the custom-designed culture with added antibiotics to which *Campylobacter* was resistant. By further creating a low oxygen, warmer environment, the microbe grew easily. After learning to culture it, Skirrow then conducted a study in a nearby medical practice and found the organism in 7 percent of the patients with diarrhea and in none of the controls. Once the problem of isolating the bacterium was solved—a special medium now makes culturing *Campylobacter* much easier—researchers around the world began finding it virtually everywhere. But perhaps it is not simply being cultured more easily and more often, but actually is more prevalent than before. There are many reasons to believe that the way we are raising poultry today encourages this pathogen.

Outbreaks have also been reported from drinking raw milk and from eating undercooked hamburger. In recent years infections have been associated with contaminated milk bottles in England (where they still deliver milk), when birds pecked off the shiny foil caps and in the process contaminated the milk. (Perhaps they had picked up the bug while looking for worms in cattle or poultry waste.)

It has also caused illness in hikers who drank water from streams, and several widespread outbreaks have been associated with contaminated municipal water supplies. One of the first was in Bennington, Vermont, but a far larger outbreak took place in the tiny town of Greenville, Florida. Of the town's 1,096 residents, 865 became ill, some desperately so. The source of the infection was linked to the town's water supply, which had apparently become contaminated by wild birds at a time when the prechlorinator was not functioning properly. Where had the birds picked up the infection? The environmental sources are probably many, but a poultry farm was nearby, which might well have been a source.

Of all the possible ways of contracting campylobacteriosis (the name of the illness caused by the bacterium), by far the most likely source in the food supply is poultry. Widespread outbreaks on two college campuses have linked illnesses to either undercooking or poor handling of raw chicken in the kitchen, where cross-contamination or direct contamination has occurred.

Symptoms of infection with *Campylobacter* usually begin within seven days after exposure and last about a week, although it *can* last 10 days. Generally the infection causes watery or "sticky" diarrhea that may become bloody, and it is generally accompanied by fever, malaise, abdominal pain, and sometimes nausea. Usually the infection ends on its own, but in some severe cases a physician may prescribe an antibiotic. Treatment with erythromycin or a fluoroquinolone reduces the length of time that individuals shed the bacteria in their stools, but whether it is needed is a decision to be made with the advice of a physician.

If all a *Campylobacter* infection did was produce intense but short-lived gastrointestinal symptoms, it would be unpleasant enough, but there can be rare, long-term consequences from the illness. It can cause reactive arthritis, a debilitating syndrome that can sometimes lead to chronic arthritis. It can cause Reiter's syndrome, which is characterized by arthritis, urethritis, and conjunctivitis combined. And it is one of several infections that *can* lead to Guillain-Barré syndrome, a serious illness characterized by progressive paralysis that occurs after an individual's immune system is triggered to attack the body's own nerves. This is an illness that usually requires intensive care. Recent studies indicate that from 38 percent to 46 percent of cases of Guillain-Barré follow recognized infection with *Campylobacter jejuni,* but the syndrome occurs in only one in every 1,000 cases of campylobacteriosis. Infection with the pathogen has also been associated with meningitis, convulsions, bacteremia, and less frequently, miscarriage.

These are all debilitating souvenirs that can substantially alter the lives of those who have a chance encounter with this bug. While it doesn't often cause death, it certainly can. The CDC estimates that between 200 and 730 people die of *Campylobacter* infection in the United States each year, and it considers that figure an underestimate. (When these numbers are added to the illnesses and deaths attributed to *Salmonella,* also frequently linked to poultry, the tendency of health-conscious Americans to make chicken the centerpiece of their diet becomes somewhat ironic.)

One fact that has turned up in various studies is that people can acquire immunity to *Campylobacter.* In underdeveloped countries such as Pakistan, says Dr. Martin Blaser, a *Campylobacter* expert at Vanderbilt University, children get infected early and, if they survive, appear to develop immunity. An outbreak in the United States revealed a similar pattern when a fraternity had an outing at a farm and drank raw milk. The clue was that not everyone who drank the milk got sick—the exceptions being the farm family, who always drank the milk, and those fraternity members with "prior raw-milk experience." It may well be that our higher sanitation standards when combined with the concentrated exposure we receive from some food products create a problem that is new. But intentionally exposing our children to *Campylobacter* to see which one survives and which one does not is obviously not an option.

Getting rid of *Campylobacter* in the environment is not going to be easy. Manure from any animal is potentially a major source of pathogens, especially now that farming is intensified, the population is increasing, and more and more individuals are eating more and more meat—which translates into a huge increase of food animals. (While the number of vegetarians is growing, individual consumers of animal protein are eating more of it, more frequently, than ever before.) When researchers in the Netherlands looked at the problem of *Campylobacter* from poultry waste water, they found it to be an important environmental source of contamination, and this was after the water had gone through a sewage treatment plant. Thus not only animal waste but human waste from individuals infected with *Campylobacter* has the potential to provide a "constant flow of this pathogen into the environment," said the researchers.

Fortunately Swedish poultry producers have found a way, if not to eliminate *Campylobacter*, then to reduce it considerably by using the same simple but effective means they employ to produce *Salmonella*-free chickens. Clean feed, clean houses, clean water, less stress, elimination of antibiotic use except for treatment of disease, and careful transportation all can reduce infection in the birds. Other studies have shown a reduction on poultry that was air chilled during processing rather than water chilled. (*Campylobacter* does not like dry surfaces.) But getting rid of *Campylobacter* may be virtually impossible, and reducing it is not going to be easy. There are no quick fixes.

Campylobacter jejuni

A rod-shaped, gram-negative bacterium that moves freely using flagella and has a pronounced preference for a warm, reduced-oxygen environment.

Illness: Campylobacteriosis

Signs and symptoms: Diarrhea that may turn bloody or may contain mucus; fever; malaise; nausea and vomiting

Onset time: Within a week of exposure, usually 1 to 4 days

Average duration of illness: 4 to 7 days with rare cases lasting 10 days

Severity: Mild to moderate

Fatality rate: 0.05 percent

Foods at particular risk of contamination: Raw meats, unpasteurized milk, contaminated water

Nonfood sources: Kittens and puppies

Treatment: Treatment with erythromycin or a fluoro-quinolone can reduce the duration of the infection, but a decision as to whether treatment is needed should be made with the advice of a physician. Antibiotics are generally not recommended. A supportive regime of fluid maintenance or replacement is preferred.

SALMONELLA

In November 1997 reports began appearing in local newspapers of what seemed to be a growing outbreak of foodborne disease in St. Mary's County, Maryland. An older woman had become seriously ill, then had died, and some three dozen other people were hospitalized. There was a classic feel to the outbreak; all of the people had been to an annual church supper. But within days the number of sick people would climb dramatically. Eventually more than 700 of the 1,400 people who had attended the annual dinner in Chaptico, a small town about 65 miles south of Baltimore, would become ill. The suspect food: stuffed hams—from the same recipe that had been used for 50 years. What had gone wrong? Ironically, in the interest of food safety the hams had not been boiled at parishioners' homes, as in the past, but at a commercial seafood distributor. Investigators surmised that the heat used in cooking had not been enough to penetrate all the hams and kill the *Salmonella* microbes lurking in the stuffing. (Had they been prepared as in years past at parishoners' homes, it would have been unlikely that all the hams would have been improperly cooked, and the outbreak would have been smaller. Mass production undertaken in the interest of food safety can backfire because mistakes can have much larger consequences.)

Salmonella is a name that rolls pleasantly off the tongue. It sounds more like a type of Italian pasta than a pathogenic organism. Yet it is a large genus of bacteria, discovered more than a hundred years ago by an American scientist named Salmon, which explains the name. The microbes were undoubtedly scourges to humans long before being identified. Most people have heard of typhoid fever, an infection that begins in the lymph nodes and can enter the bloodstream, where it may infect the liver, kidneys, spleen, bone marrow, gall bladder, and sometimes the heart. It may seem an illness of the infectious past, but typhoid fever still afflicts 200 to 400 people each year in the United States. It comes from infection with the bacterium *Salmonella typhi*.

Large outbreaks of typhoid fever still—rarely—occur from domestic sources of infection. In 1982, 72 people with typhoid fever in San Antonio, Texas, had their infections traced to food that had been contaminated by infected food-service workers at a tortilla restaurant. Like the infamous Typhoid Mary of the early 1900s, the workers themselves had no symptoms, a strong reminder that asymptomatic carriers of the typhoid bacillus are still among us and have the potential to be a community problem.

Salmonella is such a large genus that it can be divided into groups and then into species and serotypes, many of which act on the body in different ways. The unfortunately all-too-familiar intestinal upset caused by infection with certain strains is called *Salmonella* gastroenteritis. It makes about 2 million to 4 million people sick each year in the United States. About 200,000 are likely to see a doctor. Many of these are hospitalized, and the infection kills as many as 2,000 annually. The diarrhea, fever, and abdominal cramps that are typical usually develop 12 to 72 hours after infection, and the illness lasts from four to seven days. While most people recover on their own, and antibiotics are not generally recommended at this stage, since they could make matters worse, in some the infection can spread from the intestines to the bloodstream and then to other organs in the body. Unless the patient is promptly treated with antibiotics at this point, the level of infection may well be fatal. Others less seriously infected still may be left with unpleasant reminders in the form of lingering disabilities. Long after the initial episode is over, a few victims may be left with Reiter's syndrome, which is characterized by joint pain, urethritis, and irritation (conjunctivitis) in the eyes, or a condition called reactive arthritis. Both of these maladies can be extremely debilitating and can last for months or even years, sometimes becoming chronic arthritis.

Salmonella bacteria are commonly found on raw animal products, especially poultry of all sorts, and more and more frequently these days, in eggs. Most salmonellae dwell contentedly in the intestinal tract of farm animals, birds, and reptiles, generally without causing these hosts too much harm. Water or food intended for humans may become contaminated with fecal material from these sources— say, during the slaughtering process of food animals—or from infected humans who handle food. Outbreaks have been linked to cheese, poultry, beef, lamb, cantaloupe, milk, yeast, chocolate, beef jerky, and eggs. *Salmonella* has contaminated powdered milk products and infant formula as well as cake mixes. Most famously, perhaps, is the stuffing in turkeys that becomes contaminated and is not sufficiently heated during roasting to destroy the bacteria. Reported cases of salmonellosis increase immediately after holidays when people traditionally eat stuffed turkey. For some time public health warnings have focused on changing cooking habits to eliminate this risk.

Any prepared food, whether made commercially or in the home, has the potential to become the source of infection if it is contaminated and then not reheated enough to destroy the bacteria. Contaminated prepared foods can look and smell fine, so diners can't rely on their noses to tell them what could make them sick.

The egg is an exception to the problem of foods that become contaminated during processing. *Salmonella enteritidis,* which has to be given credit for being an especially clever and opportunistic strain of an especially clever and opportunistic group of bacteria, has found a way to get into the ovary of the chicken. Thus today an egg has the potential to arrive prepackaged with the pathogen inside. Since contaminated eggs served raw or less than thoroughly cooked can transmit infection (and all eggs must now be considered potentially contaminated), many cooking traditions must be revised. Public health efforts now focus on changing how we cook eggs. Among the old favorites now considered too risky to consume: soft-cooked eggs of any sort, boiled, poached, lightly scrambled, or sunny-side up; Caesar salad; mousses; meringue pies; many types of cake frosting; sauces such as béarnaise and hollandaise; homemade mayonnaise; eggnog; and homemade ice cream. Anything containing raw eggs, in other words, that isn't cooked enough to kill the bacteria could make you sick.

Even processed products may become contaminated with *Salmonella*. Large outbreaks have occurred when pasteurized milk was either inadvertently combined with unpasteurized milk or contaminated in some other way. One of the largest outbreaks ever recorded occurred in 1994 in commercial ice cream. Cases were first noticed in Minneapolis. When the state health department investigated, they found that eating Schwan's ice cream was the common thread among the sick. Since it was the *Salmonella enteritidis* strain common to eggs, that was assumed to be the source. But company officials were puzzled, since their recipe didn't include eggs. What had happened, investigators later discovered, was that the trucks that transported the ice cream premix had back-hauled raw, liquid eggs and had not been completely cleaned between loads.

What was interesting about the outbreak from the public health standpoint was that it demonstrated how a mass-produced and widely distributed product could cause a new kind of widespread outbreak, one that differed considerably from the old model, like the ham at the church supper. When investigators looked closely at the outbreak, they were able to estimate that 224,000 people in 48 states had actually been made ill, but because *Salmonella* cases are now so common and because the cases were scattered, few states realized what was going on. The company now has its own trucks and, as a backup, pasteurizes the ice-cream premix again at its plant before it is used to make ice cream. But people who assumed that commercial ice cream was a product guaranteed not to make them sick have to think again.

In the spring of 1998 more than 650 cases of salmonellosis spread across Canada. They were traced to packaged cheese snacks mainly intended for children. Like the Schwan's ice cream outbreak, the common strain of *Salmonella* and the random cases—typical of infection from a mass-produced product—meant that recognizing the outbreak as one from a single source was delayed. Officials at the CDC were alerted to look for cases among U.S. tourists returning from Canada, but none was ever reported.

New *Salmonella* serotypes appear with some regularity, and individual members of the species were once given names related to the illnesses they caused; now the names, such as *Salmonella minneapolis* or *S. arizonea,* often relate to the geographical area in which the strain was first isolated. While a person with salmonellosis doesn't usually care which serotype of the bacterium is causing distress, it can be very important in spotting an outbreak from, say, a widely distributed mass-produced food product. If a number of cases pop up from an unusual serotype, there is a good chance they come from the same source. If the product is spotted, it can be withdrawn, hopefully before it causes more trouble. In the summer of 1998, 118 cases of salmonellosis in 11 different states causing 40 hospitalizations were linked quickly to a single brand of toasted oat breakfast cereal precisely because the strain, *Salmonella agona,* was an unusual one. The company instituted a massive recall and began an investigation to determine how a toasted product could have become contaminated, and consumer confidence in food safety dropped yet another notch. Little reported by the press was a subsequent analysis by a trade association that linked *Salmonella agona* to animal-protein feed ingredients, such as fish and feather meal. The bacterium, their researchers indicated, had taken a spore form that survived toasting only to revive in milk. How this particular strain, previously found in animal feed made with fish meal, came to be on toasted cereal is still not clear.

The CDC has been monitoring *Salmonella* for over thirty years, keeping track of which strains are causing more human disease and which are causing less. The prevalence of certain strains tells us more about our society and culture, even about how we grow and distribute our foods, than one might imagine. The agency watched with a mixture of horror and fascination as cases of *Salmonella enteritidis* rose dramatically in the 1980s, first on the East Coast and now throughout the United States. It is now the single most frequently isolated strain.

Methods currently being used to raise both broiler chickens and laying hens have been implicated or hinted at in various scientific studies as bearing some responsibility. Clearly, putting 70,000 closely bred birds into a house where they are subjected to various forms of stress (such as crowding and antibiotics in feed) and exposing them to sources of infection in feed and water as well as from rodents is to establish ideal conditions for the spread of disease among them. When it is an infection that does not harm the poultry, producers have little incentive to clean up the process. Given the difficulty of tracing an illness in a human back to the hen responsible, few producers feel any pressure to change the system.

It was once thought unlikely that infections in food animals could be directly transmitted to the humans who consumed them. Now we know differently, and the stakes are getting higher. Recently a *Salmonella* strain highly resistant to most antibiotics was demonstrated to have been transmitted from animals to humans, and the link between antibiotic use in animals and the multiresistant strains that are now making humans sick is no longer seriously disputed.

Salmonella typhimurium DT104 was first reported in the United Kingdom in 1984 and is currently the second most common *Salmonella* strain causing human disease there. Illnesses in the UK have been traced to contact with farm animals and eating chicken, pork sausages, meat paste, and beef. The illnesses were serious. Forty-one percent of the patients were hospitalized, and of 195 culture-confirmed cases, 10 (5 percent) died. The fatality rate for other non-typhoid *Salmonella* infections is usually around 0.1 percent.

The microbe itself has been isolated from an assortment of animals and has been transmitted from both cattle and sheep directly to humans. Exactly what conditions it prefers and why it is now in the environment are questions researchers are attempting to answer. One thing is certain: It is an environmental problem, and something we are doing is helping to create a niche in which the microbe feels very comfortable.

The first sign that this bug had spread to the United States came in 1996 when 19 of the 32 students in a small elementary school in rural east-central Nebraska became ill with fever, vomiting, nausea, diarrhea, and in three cases, bloody diarrhea. Some of the children tested positive for the new serotype.

In July and August of 1996 the CDC's Public Health Laboratory Information System (PHLIS) found that in 29 states reported cases of *Salmonella* typhimurium (all strains) had increased substantially. It is now second only to *Salmonella* enteritidis in the frequency of reporting. But in the Nebraska outbreak the children were found to be infected with the DT104 strain of *Salmonella* typhimurium, and it was strikingly resistant to a broad range of antibiotics, including ampicillin, chloramphenicol, streptomycin, sulfonamides, and tetracycline. Investigators wondered how much of the increase they were seeing in *Salmonella* typhimurium actually came from DT104.

How did the strain acquire its broad pattern of antibiotic resistance? Researchers in the UK pointed to the use of antibiotics in animals. DT104 in the UK was, by 1996, showing resistance to trimethoprim and fluoroquinolones, both of which were used by veterinarians. After enrofloxacin was licensed for veterinary use in 1994, the number of *Salmonella* isolates from humans that were resistant to that antibiotic began to increase accordingly. It seems clear now that what is done to animals will affect humans, almost without a pause. Yet in the United States the FDA approved the use of fluoroquinolones in 1995 for poultry flocks infected with *E. coli*.

After the Nebraska cases epidemiologists kept their ears to the ground for more outbreaks from DT104. They didn't have to wait long. There were several small clusters, then in May 1997 the calves at the Heyer Hills Farm in Franklin County, Vermont, began getting sick.

The farm is in Northern Vermont in an area where the lush hills and mountains beyond create a landscape of picture-book loveliness. Take a back country road and dairy farms appear at the rate of about one a mile. Marjorie Heyer's big yellow farmhouse sits back from the road, wearing an American flag with the dignity of a dowager.

Marjorie is a widow, but not long ago her daughter Cynthia Hawley moved in with her. Cynthia, herself widowed by a farm accident, had recently sold out to move back home after 12 years of running a dairy farm alone. Her mother's farm is run by her two brothers, who live close by with their families. Cynthia took care of the calves and was especially fond of one she called Evita. When it got sick—and Cynthia could see that it was very sick, with gaunt, sunken eyes—she did everything she knew how to do, then called on her friend, the local veterinarian, Milton Robison. He suspected *Salmonella,* something calves usually fight off by themselves, and treated the animals with an antibiotic, but first Evita, then the other calves, died. Then several older cows and the farm family began getting sick. Nicholas Heyer, a nephew, was the first. His doctor put him on Bactrim, an antibiotic that combines trimethoprim and sulfamethoxazole.

Looking back, Dr. Robison shakes his head. He had thought to warn the children to stay out of the barn, but he had forgotten that, like most dairy-farm families, they drank their own raw milk. Soon five or six other people on the farm, all of whom had been drinking the milk, came down with the infection. All of them were treated with Bactrim except for Cynthia, who is allergic to sulfa drugs. She was given another antibiotic, and the result is evidence of why antibiotic treatment at this stage can be a very bad idea.

Cynthia had not drunk the milk, but she had tended the sick calves. She thought she had escaped infection, but on May 16 she too became ill. Her illness was first severe, then she got better, then much, much worse. In hindsight the antibiotic she was given was probably the reason. It didn't touch the resistant bacteria but wiped out all the competition that had been keeping it in some kind of check. The pain, she remembers, was unbelievable: "I can't begin to tell you how many times I was up during the night. I couldn't keep a thing down." She was shocked to find her symptoms—watery, bloody diarrhea—very like those of the calves that had died. When her mother insisted on taking her to the hospital, she told the emergency room nurse, "I've got *Salmonella.*" The nurse was bemused. "Let us do the diagnosing," Cynthia remembers her saying. Cynthia, of course, was right. Admitted to the hospital, her condition grew ever more serious as the infection spread to her blood. Her physicians were mystified as to why the antibiotic wasn't working. Groggily watching television in her room, she saw a report of a new multiresistant *Salmonella* strain that had been causing illnesses in England and knew instinctively it was what she had. Almost simultaneously, tests done at Cornell University on animal samples from the dead calves revealed that she was right. *Salmonella* typhimurium DT104 was the culprit. Further tests showed Cynthia was infected as well.

By 1997 the CDC was discovering that DT104 represented 10 percent of the *Salmonella* cases they were looking at. In England matters were more serious. The infection was killing 40 percent of the cattle that became infected, and 36 percent of infected humans ended up in the hospital, double the number of most foodborne illnesses.

When her doctor realized what they were dealing with, Cynthia Hawley was given a fluoroquinolone called ofloxcin. It saved her life. But the approval and use of fluoroquinolones in animal rearing means that yet another "antibiotic of last resort" may become useless as the bacteria develop resistance to it. The strong resistance most food producers have made to ending the use of antibiotics in food animals is certain now to be countered by greater pressure from both public health officials and the public alike.

In May of 1998 the *New England Journal of Medicine*'s lead article was on the emergence of multi-drug-resistant *Salmonella enterica* typhimurium DT104, and the link was made to the role of agriculture in the development of this new strain. It was important, the authors said, to find the source of this multi-drug-resistant strain and address the association between the use of the antibiotics in food animals and the growing emergence of these infections. "Prudent use of antimicrobial agents in farm animals and more effective disease prevention on farms are necessary to reduce the dissemination of five-drug-resistant typhimurium DT104 and to slow the evolution of resistance to additional agents in this and other strains of *Salmonella*." The gauntlet had been tossed down before agribusiness and the federal regulatory agencies, but was anyone listening?

Salmonella

Salmonella is a rod-shaped, non-spore-forming, and motile (although there are nonmotile exceptions) gram-negative bacterium.

Illness: Salmonellosis

Signs and symptoms: Nausea, vomiting, abdominal cramps, diarrhea (occasionally bloody) fever, headache. Chronic consequences may include arthritic symptoms 3 to 4 weeks after the onset of acute symptoms.

Onset time: 12 to 72 hours after infection

Average duration of illness: 4 to 7 days

Severity: Moderate to severe

Fatality rate: 0.1 percent, except with the DT104 strain, where it may be as high as 5 percent.

Foods at particular risk of contamination: Just about any food you can think of has the potential either to arrive in the kitchen contaminated or to be contaminated in processing. *Salmonella* can frequently be found in raw animal products such as meat, poultry, milk, and eggs. It has also been found on occasion in chocolate, shrimp, frog legs, yeast, coconut, sauces and salad dressing, cake mixes, cream-filled desserts and toppings, dried gelatins, peanut butter, ice cream, and cocoa. Fresh fruits and vegetables can be contaminated, and recent outbreaks have been traced to cantaloupe, tomatoes, fruit soups, and sprouts. Outbreaks have now been traced to processed foods such as dry cereal and cheese snack packs. *Salmonella* typhimurium DT104 has been traced to the consumption of raw milk.

Nonfood sources: People can also acquire *Salmonella* from petting infected dogs, cats, or especially reptiles. Baby turtles were once a major source of infection, and their sale is regulated. Now infections from lizards and salamanders are climbing as these animals become more popular pets.

Treatment: Often the illness resolves itself and doesn't require treatment unless the patient becomes severely dehydrated or the infection spreads from the intestines to the bloodstream (bacteremia) or another part of the body. In some patients the diarrhea is severe enough to require hospitalization for rehydration, and if the infection spreads to other parts of the body, it can be fatal unless the patient is treated at once with antibiotics, such as ampicillin, gentamicin, trimethoprim/sulfamethoxazole, or ciprofloxacin Says the CDC, "Unfortunately some *Salmonella* bacteria have become resistant to antibiotics, largely as a result of the use of antibiotics to promote the growth of feed animals." The DT104 strain can still be treated with ciprofloxacin, but that may only be a matter of time. The strain in England is ciprofloxacin-resistant. The delay may be that the veterinary use of fluoroquinolones was only approved in the United States in 1995 and only for poultry; the resistant strain has not yet appeared in poultry in the United States.

E. COLI O157:H7

Larry and Rita Bernstein and their three daughters, Samantha, Chelsea, and Haylee, live in pleasant, affluent, suburban Wilton, Connecticut, where Larry is a financial planner and Rita is a stay-at-home mom. In June 1996 Rita became ill with severe diarrhea, but within 24 hours she had recovered. A day later her youngest daughter, Haylee, who had just had her third birthday, came into her parent's room at around 3 A.M. feeling unwell. Rita took her into their bed.

Their oldest daughter, Samantha, 10, planned to leave for camp that next morning, and Chelsea, 7, had planned to go along for the ride. When Chelsea begged off making the trip, Rita knew something was wrong. Later both younger children began vomiting and having frequent diarrhea.

At first Rita wasn't too worried. "Just a bug; something going around," she thought.

When it continued through the night and into the next day, the Bernsteins took the children to their family doctor. The advice: keep up the fluids. But the girls didn't improve. Discussing the children's illness with a friend, Rita was reminded that she had recently taken the girls to a fast-food restaurant. The friend wondered if they had *E. coli* O157:H7 infection, a terrifying thought. Rita had heard, with the rest of the country, of the huge Jack in the Box outbreak in 1993, when more than 700 people became seriously ill and four died.

With no improvement, she and Larry took the children back to the doctor, who warned them to keep an eye out for blood in the children's stools. There *was* some in Haylee's stool, nothing dramatic, but by Sunday afternoon Haylee was so lethargic she fell asleep on the dining-room floor; when she was awake, she was so restless and uncomfortable that Rita could do nothing to comfort her. They took the girls to the hospital that night and both were admitted for dehydration. After tests, the diagnosis was just what Rita had feared most: infection with *E. coli* O157:H7.

"My first thought was that it was fatal and that I would lose both of them."

Chelsea remained hospitalized for three days, getting fluids intravenously. She would recover completely. But Haylee, the doctor told Rita and Larry, very likely had something called hemolytic uremic syndrome (HUS). He advised transferring her to a larger hospital where she would get specialized care.

"Great," thought Rita. "They can fix this, whatever it is."

She had no idea that Haylee would begin a horrifying roller-coaster ride that would last 14 weeks, taking their tiny daughter to the point of death several times as the toxins produced by the bacteria raced through her small body's circulatory system, shredding cells, clogging the kidneys, and damaging other organs in a vicious cascade. There is no treatment for *E. coli* O157:H7 infection, no cure for HUS. Physicians can only support the body in every possible way as it does battle with a terrifying, powerful, and unrelenting enemy. Haylee's blood would be cleaned with hemodialysis, a process that took three and a half hours every other day for more than a month. She would suffer retinal hemorrhages, pneumonia, and rectal prolapse. When she did leave the intensive care unit, she began convulsing and had to be returned. Her long hair would be shaved, and she would have brain surgery when the toxin attacked that organ as well, causing "a bleed the size of a tennis ball in her tiny brain," remembers Rita.

Haylee survived, with what are called, with deep irony, "souvenirs." Her eyes are permanently damaged, as may be her kidney function. Barring a miracle, the Bernsteins—and Haylee—will be reminded of the experience for the rest of their lives. But the culprit wasn't in the fast-food hamburgers. It was likely in a mixture of baby salad greens. There were 35 cases of infection from E. coli O157 in the area at that time, says Rita, and the health department traced 21 of them to the salad mix. Rita had been serving it to her family daily.

The cases were startling to public health officials. The E. coli O157:H7 bacteria are sometimes found in healthy cattle, and the bacteria can get onto beef when the animal's fecal material or gut contents contaminate the meat, usually during the slaughtering process. Most cases have been linked, either directly or indirectly, to hamburger because the grinding process spreads the bacteria throughout the product.

Hamburger was very likely what made Nancy and Tom Donley's son sick. The Donleys live on the north side of Chicago in a neighborhood they picked because they wanted children. Alexander Thomas Donley, or "Alex" as they called him, was born ten months after their marriage in 1986. He was healthy, and as he grew, a loving and tender child. In love with everything about being a mother, Nancy told her own mom, "This is what life's all about." But in 1993 both she and Tom lost their jobs. Nancy was the first to find work, and Tom stayed home with Alex, then six and a half. On the July 14 he called Nancy at work to tell her that Alex was complaining of a bad tummy ache and diarrhea.

Nancy came home and found Alex curled up in pain. He slept in his parents' bed that night, and in the morning, with no improvement in his discomfort, they took him to their pediatrician.

"There was something wrong with his blood," says Nancy, who admits she can't recall the medical jargon. "We took him to Children's Memorial Hospital and he was admitted right away."

Thus would begin a dreadful tale that five years later Nancy cannot relate without emotion flooding her voice. She remembers Alex, a tiny figure pushing his tall IV frame when he could still walk, struggling to the bathroom to use the toilet. Helping him, she was horrified to look down and find the bowl filled with blood and mucus. She thought to herself, "He's going to die." Things deteriorated quickly. "He hemorrhaged and hemorrhaged," she remembers. "He had neurological problems, he couldn't control his eyes, and there were tremors."

The doctors recognized that Alex had HUS and told Nancy that there was no cure, nothing they could do except support his body as it engaged in a desperate battle. He was visibly swelling. He was having delusions. She came back from a break to find the medical team had drilled holes in his head to insert shunts to drain the fluid from his swelling brain. The horror of watching her child go downhill so quickly is still painfully vivid. "He was hooked up to everything imaginable. Then his lung collapsed, and they put a huge hole in his side to insert a tube. He had a seizure and they called 'Code Blue.' Then they put him on a respirator." It had been only four days since his diarrhea began.

Like so many families, the Donleys then faced the terrible question of when to cut off the life support. There were no brain waves. Doctors told them he would not recover. Alex Donley died on July 18, just five days after he had taken ill. The staff was in shock, remembers Nancy. They had worked so hard, but there was nothing else they could do.

"When the autopsy report came in," says Nancy, "we just couldn't believe the destruction to his body. Portions of his brain were liquefied. They couldn't even get a tissue sample to make a slide. His bowel was gangrenous; his heart was double the normal size and his lungs coated with a strange fluid. We asked about donating organs, but there was nothing to donate except his corneas."

The species E. coli is probably the most common bacterium in the world. They are found in the guts of both humans and animals, where they are usually harmless or sometimes even helpful. It is the genus of bacteria about which researchers know the most. *E. coli* bacteria are used extensively in genetic research experiments both because they are so familiar and because they reproduce so rapidly—about every 22 minutes. While the infamous *E. coli* O157:H7 is now the most familiar of those that cause human disease, there are, in fact, five recognized classes of *E. coli* that are pathogenic. They are grouped according to *how* they cause disease: enteropathogenic, enterotoxigenic, enteroinvasive, enteroaggregative, and enterohemorraghic. This last is the category into which O157 falls. Because the enterotoxigenic *E. coli* strains mainly cause infections in travelers in underdeveloped countries, and the other classes rarely cause illness in the United States, this chapter will focus on O157 and touch briefly on the other toxin-producing *E. coli* that produce bloody diarrhea.

In 1993 testing for *E. coli* O157:H7 was uncommon, and Alex was never tested, but today it is well known that the bacterium is responsible for about 85 percent of HUS cases. (*Shigella,* another foodborne bacterium that produces the virulent toxin, and several other pathogens are responsible for the rest.) The hospital carefully went over everything the Donleys had eaten before Alex had gotten sick, and once again the finger of suspicion pointed toward the frozen ground-beef patties they often served. But nothing could be proved. Alex Donley became another tragic sporadic case that left everyone with more questions than answers. That is quite typical, but in numerous other instances hamburgers have been identified, both epidemiologically and by finding the same strain of the pathogen in both the victim and the meat.

"This wasn't just a statistic. His death didn't just affect us," says Nancy. "It has had a ripple effect among our friends, family, his school and playmates, and even the community. Life can never be the same."

Today she works, because she feels sure Alex would want her to, for a group called Safe Tables Our Priority (S.T.O.P.), which supports victims and their families. They have lobbied, with the medical community, to make the reporting of *E. coli* O157:H7 mandatory, and today, in most states, it is, although some remain resistant.

The characteristics of infection with O157 are much like those Rita Bernstein and Nancy Donley describe. The first sign is usually nonbloody diarrhea. In many it develops no further. There is intense cramping, such as Alex experienced, so severe that women often describe it as similar to labor pains. Fever isn't typical—it is more common if the infection becomes severe. Those who develop bloody diarrhea are usually the only ones who seek medical care. About 50 percent of patients have vomiting along with diarrhea. The infection may last no longer than a week. Intense lethargy is often reported in those who develop HUS. Even cases that do not deteriorate into HUS may leave patients with damage that can include perforated bowel, bowel necrosis, and even lung, heart, and nervous system damage. Unfortunately, the infection is often misdiagnosed, because it looks so much like other disorders, such as appendicitis, intussusception, inflammatory bowel disease, and ischemic colitis. Patients who are misdiagnosed may even have unnecessary surgery.

Infection with *E. coli* O157:H7 is more prevalent than the public may imagine since it is usually only the largest outbreaks that make the paper. In fact, the CDC estimates that as many as 20,000 people in the United States may be infected each year. While the death rate from E. coli 0157 is difficult to establish with certainty, and some authorities indicate a higher figure, the CDC's expert, Dr. Patricia Griffin, puts the number at around a hundred. The infection is now the chief cause of kidney failure in children in North America.

As to how best to avoid infection, the chief message to consumers has been to cook hamburgers thoroughly. In fact, cooking has been the generally recommended solution to outbreaks from other food sources. But ever more frequently illnesses are being caused by foods one doesn't expect to cook. In 1995 an outbreak of illnesses was caused by bottled fresh apple juice, and again the solution seemed to be the application of heat. Pasteurization might spoil the taste and reduce the nutritional content of juice, but it could kill the bacteria, and for people who wanted to be safer, it was an option. The government considered whether it should require pasteurization for all juices, even as demand was growing for bottled fresh juices, which many consumers considered healthier. Today juices must indicate if they are unpasteurized and point out the dangers.

The baby salad greens that caused the infections in Connecticut weren't meant to be cooked. Nor was their processing well regulated. Epidemiologists had identified lettuce as a possible source of contamination before, but now there was no doubt. Nor did consumers expect to have to cook alfalfa sprouts, which caused outbreaks of O157 infection in both Virginia and Michigan in 1997. You could cook the dickens out of your hamburger meat and be pretty sure you were safe, but how thoroughly did you need to wash your lettuce to be sure it was pathogen-free? Were there any guarantees at all?

Before the 1993 Jack in the Box outbreak, most Americans had never heard of E. coli O157:H7. In fact, it was only identified as a cause of human diarrheal disease in 1982 after an outbreak from McDonald's hamburgers in the Medford, Oregon, area and later in Traverse City, Michigan. Investigators from the Centers for Disease Control and Prevention (CDC) matched the bacterial strain in patients with the strain found in quality-control samples the company had held. Between 1982 and 1993 there were numerous outbreaks, and from each one the epidemiologists learned more about the character of the new threat to food safety. There were also sporadic, isolated cases, and in many, perhaps most, the specific food bearing the culprit was never identified. Later studies showed the cases were probably from mass-distributed hamburger, and the random appearances of the illnesses meant that no clear outbreak was ever spotted. There were also outbreaks from apple cider, from contaminated drinking and swimming water, from person-to-person transfer, and from foods tainted by cross-contamination in the kitchen or in packing. All the cases could be traced back to contamination of food or water with animal or human waste. In the case of the Bernsteins' salad greens, an investigation once again indicated that cattle waste had probably contaminated the water in which the lettuce had been washed. It looked clean. Rita Bernstein doesn't remember if she washed it thoroughly or even if she washed it at all; seemingly clean vegetables lull consumers into complacency. In fact, a restaurant owner admits that he and many other restaurants he knows about never rewash purchased prewashed salad greens.

Investigators had been surprised by the new pathogen in 1982; as they tracked the growing number of outbreaks, they were startled

by its virulence. From 5 to 7 percent of those who are infected with
E. *coli* O157:H7 develop the HUS that affected Haylee Bernstein
and Alex Donley. Of those, between 3 and 5 percent die. Another
12 percent are left with conditions that may require transplants, or
leave them blind or neurologically impaired.

In one outbreak in Canada, 19 nursing-home residents died during an outbreak with 55 victims; among those who had progressed
to HUS or thrombotic thrombocytopenic purpura (TTP), the adult
version of the syndrome, which less frequently involves renal failure,
the death rate was a horrifying 88 percent. In England in 1996, the
infection killed 20 people in a single outbreak that made several
hundred ill, and in Japan, 22 died when a widespread outbreak
struck literally thousands. Around the globe, public health officials
and consumers were awakening to the new E. *coli* O157:H7 reality,
and they were finding it in anything that had come in contact with
cattle waste. Here and there were hints that it might have spread to
a natural reservoir as well. In some areas of the United States, deer
tested positive; one researcher found it in gull dung, not really surprising for these scavengers.

There is something about the idea of a *new* disease-causing organism that can hardly fail to cause excitement. New—what exactly
does that mean? Is the organism simply newly recognized? Or is it
newly causing illness because we have become, for some reason,
more susceptible? Perhaps it is genuinely new, the product of mutation, or conjugation, or genetic engineering. Both the HIV and
Ebola virus were new, and both shook our complacency about the
ability of medicine and science to cure infectious diseases even as
they intrigued and terrified. But in both these cases the microbes
had probably been around for some time, lurking in animal popula-
tions or remote forests where they did not regularly come into contact with human beings. Something we did, changes in the way we
interacted with the environment or changes in human behavior,
were likely responsible for first the contact, then the spread of these
infections.

In this case, an E. *coli* that already had the ability to attach to the
cells of the intestine seems to have picked up the ability, through
conjugation, to produce a particularly vicious toxin, Shiga toxin. It
is the same toxin produced by *Shigella*. While the E. *coli* alone can

cause diarrhea, it is the combination of the microbe and the Shiga
toxin that causes the real damage and puts O157:H7 in a new category of seriousness. Indeed, there are, according to Canadian researchers who have been tracking the toxin, over 100 *E. coli* strains
that produce the toxin. Not all, in fact very few, have been actually
linked to human disease. But some have. There have been reports
from around the world of infection from the strains O26:H11,
O111:NM, and O113:H21, and in the United States there have
been outbreaks from O104:H21. Disease specialists at the CDC
think that we will be seeing more cases of human disease from these
other shiga toxin–producing *E. coli,* and yet O157:H7 seems to
cause the most problems. That may be because it is the easiest to detect. Because it also has the unique characteristic of not fermenting
sorbitol rapidly, a fairly simple laboratory test, the sorbitol-
MacConkey, was devised early on to make identification relatively
quick and easy. The special medium is available now in most labs.
The other strains are more difficult to detect and are likely to be
overlooked unless labs are especially watching for them; most are
not.

Most strains of O157:H7 are not resistant to antibiotics, but
treating the infection with them is very controversial. There is evidence that antibiotics may make the infection worse, or that those
treated with antibiotics may be more likely to develop HUS; there
are also studies that show that patients receiving an appropriate antibiotic (one the microbe is not resistant to) had fewer cases of
HUS. But all the studies are small and the question is still open.
More studies are needed. It is definitely not a good idea to give an
antibiotic to which the bacterium might be resistant, as it might
wipe out the microbial competition in the gut, allowing *E. coli*
O157:H7 to multiply freely.

It is also counterproductive to give antidiarrheal medication, because the body must rid itself of the toxin. Cases of bloody diarrhea
should be cultured for *E. coli* O157:H7. Children and the elderly
should be watched closely for signs of dehydration and monitored
for signs of HUS or TTP.

The evidence from various studies is that it takes only a few microbes of O157 to cause infection. That means that unlike some
foodborne pathogens, person-to-person transfer is more of a prob-

lem, especially in day-care centers and nursing facilities where fecal incontinence is likely. Several outbreaks, some with fatal consequences, have occurred in such places.

The virulence of O157, and now its presence on foods usually eaten without further cooking, is presenting a confusing and discouraging picture to cooks and indeed to everyone. While there are no guarantees, it is possible to lower the risks by using appropriate food-safety strategies, and that is what we must do.

Even that strategy was undermined in the summer of 1998, when more than two dozen children became infected with the pathogen while swimming at a popular attraction, White Water, outside of Atlanta. Many became frighteningly ill and were hospitalized, sometimes for long periods, and one three-year-old child, McCall Akin, died. As if to undermine further the feelings of security of parents everywhere, something was particularly shocking about the idea of children who were enjoying themselves so innocently contracting such a frightening infection. It was only the second outbreak ever from a chlorinated pool, and the chlorine level at the facility tested below the standard. Eventually the guilty strain would be traced back to one found in hamburger produced in Florida that had been recalled because of the presence of E. coli O157:H7, and it was likely that an infected child with liquid stools had contaminated the water. But the point was made. This bug travels easily and swiftly in the environment, and while it may originate in a cow, it can occur wherever animal or human waste is spread. And that may be in new and unexpected places. McCall Akin and her family were vegetarians.

In one of the few bits of good news about this pathogen, researchers at Cornell have recently discovered that the changed diet of cattle and cows—they are being fed grain to promote growth and milk production—may be responsible for establishing the acidic conditions that favor E. coli O157. Switching these animals to hay for five days before slaughter appears to rid them of the pathogen, thus keeping it out of the slaughterhouse environment. The challenge will be making sure this is done, as the change cannot be mandated under present USDA regulatory authority, which does not extend to the farm.

While O157 (and other Shiga toxin–producing strains) is poten-

tially the most dangerous of the *E. coli* strains, there was another surprise in the summer of 1998 when 4,000 people in the Chicago
area became ill from an *E. coli* that was an enterotoxic serotype, or
ETEC. The source was potato salad made by a local deli, and the
salad was eaten at literally hundreds of parties in the Chicago area
one June weekend. What struck investigators is that ETEC is common—but not in the United States. It is a frequent cause of traveler's diarrhea in developing countries. There have been only 14
ETEC outbreaks in the United States in the last 23 years. Expect
more as the world becomes a smaller place.

E. coli O157:H7

A gram-negative bacillus. The *O* refers to the somatic, the *H*
to the flagellar, antigen. The organisms cause disease by penetrating the epithelial cells of the gut, where they release
toxin and cause tissue distruction.

Illness: Infection with *E. coli* O157:H7

Signs and symptoms: Diarrhea, often bloody; intensely
painful abdominal cramping; sometimes nausea and vomiting
or fever

Onset time: Usually 3 to 5 days, although 5 to 8 days is
not uncommon.

Average duration of illness: 3 to 7 days

Severity: Moderate to severe

Fatality rate: 2 percent

Foods at particular risk of contamination: Hamburger meat is a significant source of the bacteria. Vegetables
contaminated with cattle manure have also caused infections.
Drinking water and milk contaminated after processing have
caused outbreaks as well.

Nonfood sources: Outbreaks have been linked to contaminated swimming areas and person-to-person transmission in day-care or nursing facilities.

Treatment: Antibiotic use is very controversial with
O157 infection. It should probably be avoided unless some
compelling reason can be put forth in its favor. There are indications it can worsen the course of the illness and the risk
of complications.

SHIGELLA

There is a dirty little secret about foodborne disease, one that is often described in abstract ways to avoid the pictures that might come from speaking more directly. While contaminated food may make you sick, the contamination may have arrived, not on the food itself, but via the hands of someone who is ill and has careless bathroom habits, who doesn't wash his or her hands before preparing foods. A diner who has awakened to this reality thinks twice before ordering a salad in a restaurant, because inevitably the disturbing question of who has prepared it and whether they are good hand washers comes to mind. In fact, salad bars have become notorious as sources of foodborne infections.

One bug that is supremely comfortable with this route of transmission is *Shigella,* and most of the outbreaks it causes are by what is gently called "the fecal-oral route."

That's what happened in Michigan in 1995 when 46 people became ill with shigellosis, as infection with *Shigella* is called, after having eaten tossed salad at different outlets of a single restaurant chain. That was a sure clue for the epidemiologists who investigated, to look at the central kitchen. They found that several of the prep workers had been ill but had continued to work. The salad makers weren't following sanitation rules. Even if the salad had been kept thoroughly chilled, it could still have been a vehicle for *Shigella* because it doesn't take many microbes to make people sick—as few as 10 to 100 microbes have been shown to cause illness. *Shigella* is also a fragile organism. It is easily killed by the heat used in cooking or processing and it does not survive well in acidic foods, so most outbreaks are linked to raw or previously cooked foods contaminated either while being prepared or, in the case of cooked foods, while being stored, combined with other ingredients, or served.

An interesting aspect of the Michigan outbreak was the central kitchen. Today salads are often made somewhere other than where they are eaten, and this wasn't the first time central preparation of salad ingredients had been linked to a large outbreak. In 1985, 5,000 people in the Midland-Odessa, Texas, area became ill from chopped, bagged lettuce prepared for a Mexican restaurant chain. When investigators from the FDA carried out further research, they discovered that *Shigella sonnei* could survive in the chopped lettuce even under refrigeration. Worse, they found that the contaminated lettuce showed no signs of deterioration—nothing that would have indicated its potential to cause serious illness.

Outbreaks caused by *Shigella* have also occurred on cruise ships, where infected workers have been implicated. Potato salad was the culprit on one ship where 84 passengers were sick. Thirteen were hospitalized. Treatment with antibiotics was blamed for making the illnesses worse because the particular *Shigella* strain was multiresistant. In such situations, treating patients with an antibiotic can remove the microbial competition in the gut, giving the resistant microbes a clear playing field. The source was thought to be an infected food handler from a country where multiple-antibiotic-resistant *Shigella* is common. The CDC investigators thought the shortage of toilet facilities for the crew was a factor in the spread of the infection.

The problem of infected food handlers raises some important questions we seldom think of. How much a food handler is paid, whether he or she gets sick leave, how well he or she is trained—all these factors can have an impact on the safety of foods we eat outside the home. But we seldom give a thought to the implications of such social and economic issues on our health. Members of Congress who spend their political lives eating food prepared by others might think about this the next time they vote against raising the minimum wage. One epidemiologist at the CDC wonders how many outbreaks on cruise ships could be prevented if the crew didn't think that revealing they were ill might be cause for putting them ashore at the next port.

The ease with which humans can transmit *Shigella* to each other is due to the fact that it is carried in the guts of animals, but principally primates, making human waste the chief source. The rod-shaped bacteria can attach to and penetrate the epithelial cells that line the intestine. Once settled in they multiply within the cells and spread, a process that breaks down the cells. Some of the strains produce a vicious toxin, virtually identical to that produced by *E. coli* O157:H7. Complications of the infection can include Reiter's syndrome, reactive arthritis, and hemolytic uremic syndrome. Ulcers in the mucous lining of the intestine, rectal bleeding, and serious dehydration may result from infection. With some strains the death rate can be as high as 10 to 15 percent, especially in the elderly, infants, and the infirm. Shigellosis is very common among people with AIDS as well as non-HIV-infected homosexual men, as *Shigella flexneri* is now understood to be a sexually-transmitted infection as well.

There are four different species of the rod-shaped bacterium, and *Shigella dysenteriae* causes what is commonly called, simply, dysentery—usually in less developed countries. *Shigella sonnei* is the most common cause of dysentery in the United States, with the *Shigella flexneri* coming in second. Cases are increasing. In one two-year period between 1986 and 1988 the reported rate at which *Shigella* is isolated from stools in the United States doubled. Outbreaks of shigellosis have been linked to swimming in contaminated water, and contaminated water and ice on a cruise ship caused more than 600 illnesses in another outbreak.

Contaminated wells can also be a source. In August 1995 visitors staying at a resort motel in Island Park, Idaho, not far across the state line from Yellowstone National Park, began getting sick. They were experiencing the classic symptoms of fever, abdominal pain, and diarrhea (some with bloody stools). Cultures turned up *Shigella sonnei*. The source of illness for 82 people was eventually determined to be well water.

Investigators discovered that the water table was higher than usual because of heavy rains earlier in the year. The *Shigella* organisms had apparently spread through groundwater. The solution was to boil drinking water. The resort dug a new and deeper well. The cases stopped.

An uncommon means of transmitting *Shigella* was revealed in Europe in 1994. In June, public health officials in Sweden noticed an unusual number of cases of shigellosis, and *Shigella sonnei* was identified. The report of the cases went out over a European network that began as a means of reporting *Salmonella* but now provides a timely, on-line system for tracking other pathogens. Lettuce was a common factor in the cases. The bacterial strains were subtyped, and the information was distributed through Epinet, a system for transmitting data to districts throughout England. Public health workers throughout the British Isles were asked to look out for cases and found them. Most were linked to eating lettuce as well. The lettuce had come from the same source—Spain.

In the meantime, Sweden was discovering the same thing, as was Norway. Somehow lettuce shipped from Spain to northern Europe had effectively distributed *Shigella* microorganisms at the same time. What had caused the contamination? The investigators thought the irrigation water or the washing process was probably responsible, but the outbreak demonstrates the potential for the global food trade to cause widespread outbreaks.

"If iceburg lettuce is not washed thoroughly before consumption, contamination could be retained in the leaves," the investigators said in their report on the European outbreak. Actually, there are serious questions as to whether washing is sufficient to get rid of pathogenic microbes, but that is a matter for another chapter.

Not all the cases in northern Europe, investigators found, were related to the Spanish lettuce; in Wales some were linked to consumption of a commercially prepared ice cream or contact with children who had eaten the product. Virtually any food can become contaminated during preparation or serving, and what these outbreaks of *Shigella* illustrate is the importance of careful hygiene—basic hand washing first and foremost—on the part of food handlers. If there are truly basic rules that *Shigella* can teach for avoiding foodborne pathogens, they are that animal and human fecal material must be kept away from the food we eat, that sick workers should not be allowed to handle food, and that all produce should be careful washed before it is consumed.

Shigella

Gram-negative, nonmotile, non-spore-forming, rod-shaped bacteria. They cause disease when the organisms attach to, and penetrate, epithelial cells of the intestinal mucosa. After invasion, they multiply within the cells and spread to nearby epithelial cells, where they cause tissue destruction. Some strains produce the shiga toxin.

Illness: Shigellosis

Signs and symptoms: Diarrhea (there may be blood, pus, or mucus in the stools), abdominal pain, vomiting, fever

Onset time: 12 to 50 hours after infection is normal, but one reference says the illness may take as long as a week to show up.

Average duration of illness: 1 to 7 days

Severity: Moderate to severe

Fatality rate: 0.1 percent

Foods at particular risk of contamination: Salads, (potato, tuna, shrimp, macaroni, and chicken), raw vegetables, milk and dairy products, poultry

Nonfood sources: Person-to-person contact. Outbreaks are frequent in day-care settings.

Treatment: "Treatment with an antibiotic to which *Shigella* is susceptible decreases the duration of the illness," says the CDC, but antibiotic resistance among *Shigella* is increasing, and "it is important for the clinician to be aware of local resistance patterns." When there is a large outbreak, the physician needs to weigh the benefits of using an antibiotic against the risk of producing resistant strains of *Shigella*. In general, antibiotics should be avoided. The agency does not recommend using them as prophylactics in people who have been exposed.

OTHER IMPORTANT PATHOGENS

CYCLOSPORA CAYETANENSIS

What his mother-in-law, Jan Schar, remembers is how he looked: pale, gray, very unhealthy. Chris Clemente was clearly not feeling well and hadn't been for some time. When he was at her house for dinner he picked at his food, excused himself more frequently than he should, and seemed lethargic and out of sorts. She thought, frankly, that he had cancer. It was the worse thing she could think of and only something very serious could be making her vibrantly healthy son-in-law look and act like this. But she kept her thoughts to herself. She didn't want to be "that kind" of mother-in-law, always interfering. Days went by and there were times he seemed to be better and times he seemed worse. But he clearly wasn't well.

Her worry mounted. Then early one evening her daughter Tracy called her in a panic.

Chris seemed out of his head, speaking nonsensically. He was in a state of physical collapse, his strength gone. She had to have help quickly. Jan told her to call the rescue squad, then raced the six miles through the Virginia suburbs to their house. Chris was taken to the hospital where he was immediately admitted. His problem was that he was severely dehydrated, a symptom of which is incoherence and irrationality. His fluids were depleted, and his body salts in serious disequilibrium. Without intravenous rehydration he could have slipped into a coma and died. Doctors suspected what was the matter with Chris. It had been happening to a lot of people in the area.

In the middle of June 1997 at Wolf Trap Farm, an open-air concert hall outside of Washington, D.C., the unthinkable had occurred. A violinist with the National Symphony Orchestra got up in the middle of a performance and left the stage, compelled by an urgent call of nature. Eventually 32 members of the orchestra would become victims of the same fiercely unpleasant and ongoing intestinal illness caused by an unusual parasite. Outbreak investigators would ultimately identify more than 300 people in the area around Washington who were made ill from the same nasty intruder.

The source? Fresh basil and pesto—a flavorful ground piñon nut and basil mixture that had been made into 88 different food items at the central kitchen of a well-known area gourmet food-market chain. The orchestra members had consumed a pesto-pasta salad at a potluck dinner for retired members. Somehow *Cyclospora,* a new entrant onto the growing list of dangerous bugs, had gotten into the dish.

Cyclospora cayetanensis, a one-celled parasite, was first linked to human disease only recently when investigators looked back at an outbreak from an unknown source in 1977 in Papua New Guinea. But this organism, instead of targeting more humble foods, like the hamburger bacteria *E. coli* O157:H7, has fancier tastes, seeming to favor the haunts and foods of the better off.

In the Washington outbreak the contaminated foods reached fancy luncheons and other elegant affairs in the area and felled cor-

porate officials and NBC employees as well as the orchestra members. Over 100 sporadic cases were identified among members of
the public who simply bought expensive gourmet preparations over
the counter. Chris Clemente had picked up salads and sandwiches
from the specialty gourmet deli almost every day.

Cyclospora's entrance into the U.S. food supply was a surprise.
Travelers to exotic places had come back into the country infected
with the bug, but the first outbreak that originated in the United
States occurred at a golf course only in 1994, where the source of
the infection was thought to be contaminated portable watercool-
ers. Only three outbreaks had been identified in the United States
until the spring of 1996, when the public's strawberry days were
spoiled—with American growers suffering heavy losses—as outbreaks *seemed* to be linked to the fruit. The culprit at elegant wed-
ding receptions, bridesmaid's luncheons, and fancy restaurant
dinners was actually found not in the strawberries but in imported
raspberries from Guatemala. Consumer demand for fruits and vegetables without regard for their seasons surely play a role in the increase of infections from exotic pathogens such as *Cyclospora*.
Raspberries are ripe in July in the Massachusetts area; if you eat
them in May, you can be certain they are not local.

Imported raspberries were implicated again in the spring of 1997
in a series of outbreaks and clusters, and Chris Clemente's infection
might just as easily have come from the berries as the basil. His father often grumbled that his habit of not washing fruit before eating it was dangerous, and his father was surely right. Chris, with the
confidence that comes from being young and healthy, the arrogance, almost, of the exceptionally fit that says "my body can fend
off anything," had the habit of nibbling on raspberries, unwashed,
right from the box as he drove around in his car. Raw fruits and
vegetables are especially vulnerable to this pathogen, which may be
in water or carried by the hands of infected workers who harvest or
pack produce or prepare foods. Mesclun salad mix, an expensive
mixture of baby salad greens, turned out to be the vehicle in a *Cyclospora* outbreak on an ocean liner.

The illnesses caused—diarrhea, nausea, vomiting, and weight
loss—have often been protracted, with brief recovery, then relapses
as the pathogen goes through its life cycles.

The course of Clemente's illness was fairly typical. He found the nausea—he doesn't recall ever actually vomiting—and the diarrhea debilitating. Initially it plagued him throughout the day. Then he was better in the mornings but would have to take to his bed in the afternoons with profound fatigue. He remembers feeling severely ill, more ill than he had ever felt in his life. The bouts of diarrhea were crippling. He remembers having to stop whatever he was doing to cope. Once he was in a shopping mall and had to sit down with pain and discomfort so severe that he thought, "If the people passing by knew how horrible I felt they would call the rescue squad." He thought, frankly, that he was dying. For days he could not work. When he did return to his job, he knew he shouldn't have. He was too weak. He struggled on, as many people do who dislike admitting they are sick.

When cases first began appearing in the Washington area in the summer of 1997, the first thought of the disease detectives at the Alexandria (Virginia) Health Department was that imported produce was responsible, as it had been in the outbreak the year before. Then, after identifying products containing basil as the "vehicle," and finding no parasites on other shipments of basil, they began to look at the imported work force. Some of the foreign-born workers who prepared the basil products tested positive for *Cyclospora*. Whether they became infected in their native country, which was Guatemala, and became asymptomatic carriers (some had been in this country for eight years, although they had made trips home) or whether they picked up the pathogen taste testing the basil dishes is still not clear. What the epidemiologists do know is that they are learning more about this microbe every day as outbreaks occur more frequently. In 1997 alone there were more than 1,500 cases of *Cyclospora* infection in Americans from a pathogen no one had heard of a few years ago.

Cyclospora cayetanensis is a parasite too small to be seen without a microscope. It has a life cycle that makes it unlikely to be passed from person to person directly. According to the Centers for Disease Control and Prevention (CDC), the oocysts (egglike forms) take days to weeks under favorable environmental conditions to sporulate (release spores) and become infectious. The infection is characterized by frequent, watery, often explosive bowel movements.

Other symptoms can include loss of appetite, nausea, vomiting, substantial weight loss, bloating, increased gas, stomach cramps, muscle aches, low-grade fever, and severe fatigue. The first symptoms may take from four to ten days to develop after ingesting the parasite; the average is about a week. That makes it more difficult to identify the food vehicle—few people can remember what they ate a week before they began to develop symptoms, which may continue for days or even weeks before medical attention is sought. If the infection isn't treated, it may linger for weeks or even months, waxing and waning as the parasite goes through its life cycles. Someone may feel better for a while and then suffer a relapse. Chris Clemente felt this way, he remembers. His feelings of nausea remained for some time even after he had begun the medication and the diarrhea had ended. Six months later he had not gained back the 15 pounds he lost, even though his appetite returned. Infected individuals develop no immunity. They can become reinfected.

People who suspect they may have a *Cyclospora* infection should not treat themselves with over-the-counter medication before seeing a health-care provider. But be warned. Many health-care providers have little experience with and know next to nothing about *Cyclospora*. If stool cultures are taken and are negative, that proves nothing at all. Identifying the parasite requires special laboratory tests that are not routine, and some labs may not be set up to do them. In addition, the parasite may be difficult to identify because of its life cycle. For that reason some physicians, when they suspect *Cyclospora,* may ask for stool samples over a series of days. Of course, other organisms that cause similar symptoms should be looked for at the same time.

All of this takes time and money, something physicians may not feel they can do under the prevailing economic restraints common in the health-care field. They may do what Chris Clemente's doctor, and many health-care providers, do. Chris never had a stool examination performed. His physician just assumed, because of his pattern of consumption and his symptoms, that he was part of the outbreak. The most effective treatment appears to be a combination of two antibiotics, trimethoprim and sulfamethoxazole, sold under such brand names as Bactrim, Septra, or Cotrim. Individuals who have an allergy to sulfa drugs have a problem. No equally effective alternative drugs have been identified, but evidence is accumulating that certain antibiotics are *not* effective, a list that includes the quinolones, tinidazole, metronidazole, quinacrine, tetracycline, doxycycline, and diloxanide furoate. Sulfa-allergic patients can be treated with supportive therapy or with antibiotics that have not yet been shown to be ineffective.

Chris was treated with the recommended antibiotic combination and recovered. The problem with failing to look for the organism is that while Chris was almost certainly infected, and probably by either basil products or the raspberries, one can't be sure. He was not part of the official investigation. He was not counted among the reported cases. If his experience is typical, there may have been many more than the 300 cases reported in the Washington area. There may have been other contaminated food products than those identified in the official investigation. Perhaps the source of Chris's infection was neither raspberries nor basil products but another food that was never spotted as a vehicle. Or perhaps he didn't have *Cyclospora* infection at all but another parasite for which treatment with trimethoprim-sulfamethoxazole was effective. We will never know for sure.

Here in the United States most cases of infection with *Cyclospora* seem to appear during the spring and summer, further implicating fresh fruits and vegetables as a likely source. People of all ages are vulnerable to infection, and while traveling in developing countries is a risk factor, it is now assumed that infection can be acquired anywhere in the world. Cases have been reported with increased frequency in other countries since 1986; part of the increase is surely attributable to better techniques for detecting the parasite in stool specimens, but the growing worldwide trade in fresh fruits and vegetables is a probable cause for the increase as well. It's worth noting that no cases have been reported in individuals who ate locally grown raspberries in season. Also, after the United States called a halt to imported Guatemalan raspberries, there were no cases in 1998. Canada, which did not restrict the raspberries, did have cases.

To be certain of escaping infection, the CDC advises the following: "Based on currently available information, avoiding food or water that may be contaminated with stool is the best way to prevent infection." Unfortunately we cannot know what is on the fruits and vegetables we buy in the supermarket. The only recourse is thorough washing, and even washing may not be 100 percent effective.

Cyclospora cayetanensis

A one-celled parasite that infects the small intestine. Its complex life cycle will cause the illness to wax and wane.

Illness: Infection with *Cyclospora*

Signs and symptoms: Frequent explosive diarrhea, nausea, loss of appetite, weight loss, bloating and gas, fatigue, muscle aches, fever. Symptoms appear on average a week after infection.

Onset time: 4 to 7 days

Duration of illness: Untreated, the illness may last from a few days to a month or longer. Symptoms may come and go several times.

Severity: Varies; can be extremely debilitating

Fatality rate: Unknown

Foods at particular risk of contamination: Imported raspberries, fresh basil, and salad mix have been implicated in outbreaks, but the parasite can be transmitted by water or food contaminated with oocysts.

Treatment: See a health-care provider. Ask for a stool examination, looking for parasites; it may need to be taken several times. A combination of two antibiotics, trimethoprim and sulfamethoxazole (sold as Bactrim, Septra, or Cotrim) is effective. Those allergic to sulfa drugs are in trouble. A wide range of antibiotics have been found to be ineffective. The only recourse, other than hoping that one will eventually recover on one's own, would seem to be to try one of the antibiotics that has not yet been found ineffective.

LISTERIA MONOCYTOGENES

January 31, 1996, has to go down as a dark day for ice-cream lovers in America, for it was on that day that three separate manufacturers, distributing between them to 15 states, were advised by the FDA to recall their product because of contamination. One of these manufacturers recalled 420,000 gallons of ice cream, frozen yogurt, sorbet, and sherbet in 17 different flavors. The reason: possible or suspected contamination with *Listeria*.

Listeria refers to a genus of bacteria, of which *Listeria monocytogenes* is the strain that affects humans most frequently. It is a microorganism most people have never heard of—unless it has already made them sick—but it is a trial to the processed-food industry. The bacterium, according to the CDC, "has recently become an important public health problem in the United States."

There was a point, a veteran food scientist says, when the food manufacturers thought they had the problem of bacteria contamination in processed foods licked. Then *Listeria* appeared to plague them, and they had to start all over again.

Actually, there is nothing new about the bacteria. They have been known to infect animals since 1911. In 1929 the first human case was identified, and *Listeria* has been known for years to be a cause of meningitis. Its presence is common in the environment; it lives at the base of grasses and can be cultured from soil, silage, and other sources. Animals pick it up, then it passes through their systems, often without doing much damage. What is new is that food was, until fairly recently, never thought to be a source; it was assumed that people picked up the infection from contact with animals. But when urban dwellers began coming down with listeriosis, which is what infection with *Listeria* is called, epidemiologists knew there must be another source.

One of the first solid links of *Listeria* to food came in 1981 in Canada, when public health officials in the Maritime Provinces noticed an increase in the numbers of listeriosis cases. An investigation revealed that the sick patients were more likely to have eaten coleslaw. When the coleslaw from a patient's refrigerator was cultured, it grew *L. monocytogenes,* serotype 4b, which was the strain that had been isolated from the patient's blood. The coleslaw, which had been purchased in a container, had been prepared by a local manufacturer that had purchased carrots and cabbages from several wholesalers and many local farmers. The investigators were able to culture *L. monocytogenes* from two unopened packages of coleslaw. One of the suppliers of cabbage had a flock of sheep, two of which had died earlier of listeriosis. The cabbage had been grown in fields fertilized with both composted and fresh manure from the flock.

When the cabbage was harvested each October, it was stored in a large cold storage facility. A shipment of cabbage from this farm had been sold through a wholesaler to the coleslaw manufacturer. Forty-one people became ill during this outbreak, and of these, 18 died.

Less than 20 years later, there is now no doubt that food can be a major source of listeriosis, and when it is found in processed foods, the FDA asks that the product be recalled. Recalls happen frequently. In the past few years it has been found in prepared sandwiches, commercial potato salad and seafood salad, hummus and similar prepared deli foods, cold cooked meats, soft cheeses, uncooked hot dogs and luncheon meats, and all types of smoked fish—in short, in a lot of favorite convenience foods—the kinds of things many people grab when they haven't time to cook. *Listeria* has also been found in cut, bagged vegetables ready to go into salad or slaw.

It is a remarkably hardy organism. It can resist freezing, drying, and heat very well for a bacterium that doesn't form a spore, and it is resistant to acid conditions, salt, and nitrite. Commercial freezers stop *Listeria* from multiplying, thorough cooking will destroy it, and it can be eliminated by pasteurization. But in the food-processing environment it is known to lurk on equipment, where it can contaminate an already cooked or pasteurized product.

What makes it such a troublemaker for the processed food industry is that it is capable of growing in an atmosphere—inside the refrigerator—that usually stops or slows growth. Prepared foods that are somehow contaminated with the microbe in processing can become more dangerous to eat, although showing no sign of contamination, the longer they stay in the refrigerator. As new methods of packaging that extend refrigerator shelf life become more common, the problem of *Listeria* will probably increase.

What is curious about *Listeria* is that what might not affect one person might make another very ill indeed. Many healthy people seem unaffected by exposure, and some people carry it in their systems apparently all the time. On the other hand, pregnant women and their fetuses, as well as immune-compromised individuals and sometimes the diabetic, cirrhotic, asthmatic (who may be taking steroids—a risk factor), and those with ulcerative colitis, are especially vulnerable.

In fact, pregnant women are 20 times more likely than other healthy adults to get listeriosis, and people with AIDS are 300 times more likely to contract the infection. Otherwise healthy individuals who are taking antacids may also be at greater risk. But there are no guarantees for even the totally fit. In an outbreak in Switzerland from heavily contaminated cheese, healthy individuals did become ill, so the amount and virulence of the particular strain may play a role. Scientists are still learning about *Listeria*.

For those who do get the infection, it can be a very serious illness. The early symptoms include fever, chills, a headache, and sometimes nausea and vomiting, but this may proceed to something much more serious, such as bacteremia or meningitis. Making a diagnosis is difficult; the first symptoms may occur 12 hours after eating, but listeriosis can then take from one to six weeks to develop fully, and when it enters the bloodstream or turns into meningitis, it has a frightening 25 to 70 percent fatality rate. An outbreak in Philadelphia in 1987 produced 32 cases of listeriosis with 11 deaths.

When the victim is a pregnant woman, the mother usually survives; it is the child that is most at risk. The infection may produce early labor, and if the infant lives, it may suffer central nervous system complications, septicemia, or meningitis. A widespread outbreak affecting 142 people in California in 1985 was due to soft Mexican-style cheese and led to numerous stillbirths. Indeed the vulnerable soft cheeses include Camembert, Brie, feta, Gorgonzola, and other blue-veined cheeses, as well as the aforementioned list of popular foods. If there is one word of warning that should be issued to pregnant women—and the CDC did issue such a warning in 1992, although it received very little attention—it is to avoid entirely both the deli counter and cold cuts. If you are pregnant and insist on frequenting the deli counter, the FDA advises you to reheat all meats, including cured meats like salami and ham, before eating them. Additionally, pregnant women should eat only pasteurized dairy products and should choose hard cheeses instead of soft. All fruits and vegetables should be carefully washed. All those nice little packages of prepared foods, such as tabbouleh and the like, are best avoided. It's a shame, but the risk is simply too great. In fact, one wonders how many miscarriages might have been linked to infection with listeriosis if U.S. researchers had thought to look for the microbe. A study in France cultured *L. monocytogenes* from the placentas and/or fetuses of 1.6 percent of all pregnancies that resulted in early labor or miscarriage.

In late 1998 and early 1999 an outbreak of Listeriosis left 16 dead and caused the recall of thousands of pounds of contaminated luncheon meats and hot dogs, undermining further the public's confidence in the safety of the food supply. While large outbreaks get the press's and thus the public's attention, what is true of other foodborne pathogens is also true of *Listeria*. It generally causes sporadic illnesses that are never linked to outbreaks. Researchers at the CDC knew that the numbers from voluntary reporting were way off, and so they began looking for *L. monocytogenes* in six different regions of the United States. It was evenly distributed. When the investigators looked in the refrigerators of *Listeria* victims, they found 64 percent to contain at least one *Listeria*-contaminated food, and in 33 percent of these, the strain was the same as that infecting the sick individual. In the year examined there were 450 adult deaths and an additional 100 fetal and postnatal deaths—more than are estimated to be caused by *E. coli* O157:H7—and they consider these numbers to be conservative. Simply put, CDC experts believe that listeriosis "may well be the leading fatal foodborne infection in the United States."

Listeria monocytogenes

A ubiquitous, tough, gram-positive organism that moves using flagella. It resists heat, cold, salt, nitrate, and acidity well. It can multiply in the refrigerator with ease.

Illness: Listeriosis

Signs and symptoms: The symptoms can be flulike, with fever, fatigue, body aches, nausea, and vomiting. Sometimes only nausea and vomiting are present. Complications in pregnant women can result in miscarriage, stillbirth, or septicemia or meningitis in the newborn. In older children and adults, complications can involve the central nervous system and bloodstream. Skin contact with *L. monocytogenes* can cause localized abscesses or skin lesions.

Onset time: From a few days to 6 weeks. However, nausea and vomiting may occur as early as 12 hours after eating the contaminated food.

Average duration of illness: Days to weeks

Severity: Moderate to serious

Fatality rate: As much as 30 percent

Foods at particular risk of contamination: Soft cheeses including Mexican types, deli foods, cooked chicken, prepared sandwiches, luncheon meats, uncooked hot dogs

Nonfood sources: Contact with infected animals

Treatment: Penicillin or ampicillin

STAPHYLOCOCCUS AUREUS

If people have an idea in their heads of what foodborne disease is like, it probably mirrors staphylococcal food poisoning. The symptoms are sudden and violent, coming as few as two to four hours after eating something contaminated with the toxin that *Staphylococcus aureus* produces. One minute you are well; the next you are vomiting and retching with abdominal cramping and weakness. Along with this attractive set of symptoms (some lucky few may not experience all of them at once) may come headache, muscle cramping, and transient changes in blood pressure and pulse rate.

The source of the trouble is a gram-positive bacterium (coccus) that bunches together under the microscope like grapes or appears in pairs or short chains. What causes the illness is the highly heat-stable toxin these bacteria produce. What usually happens is that after insufficient cooking a food is held at room temperature long enough for the toxin to be produced. Or cooked foods are combined—and contaminated in the process—in a dish that is not thoroughly reheated. People were once frequently warned about egg, tuna, chicken, and potato salads; cream cakes and pies; and milk and dairy products because not only did they require handling but their ingredients were good mediums for the bacteria. Ironically it is not the mayonnaise that is the villain; it probably contains enough acid to ward off bacterial growth on its own. It is the protein foods that the bacterium seems to prefer.

It's easy to see how foods can become contaminated. *Staphylococ-*

cus bacteria exist virtually everywhere in the environment, on food equipment, on humans, and on animals. They are found in the noses and throats and on the hair and skin of 50 percent or more of healthy people. Among health-care workers the incidence is higher. Food handlers or equipment often contaminate food. Not keeping food cold or hot enough can allow the microbes to produce the toxin.

While staphylococcal poisoning has been declining in relation to other foodborne diseases, eclipsed by the emerging foodborne pathogens such as *Campylobacter, Shigella,* and *E. coli* O157:H7, cultural familiarity with the way staph poisoning works leads to confusion today. People with the classic symptoms tend to associate the illness with whatever they last ate (which is typical of foodborne illness caused by staph), and yet the newer culprits may take days to cause trouble.

A typical outbreak of *S. aureus* occurs after a reception, picnic, or institutional meal. Good examples now are somewhat dated because they are infrequent, but a garden-variety case is the one that occurred in 1983 on a cruise ship when 32 percent of the passengers became ill. The investigation implicated cream-filled pastry and poor handling.

Another large outbreak at a New Mexico country club in 1986 implicated three different foods: turkey, poultry dressing, and gravy. Cultures of the turkey and the dressing yielded *Staphylococcus* organisms. When the food handlers were tested, *S. aureus* organisms were found in some of their noses or stools. When investigators looked at how food was being handled, they found that the turkey had been left at room temperature for three hours after cooking. The same club had experienced a previous outbreak two years earlier that had been linked to burritos and tacos that had been cooked and assembled, then held at room temperature.

Food handlers and poor food-safety training were implicated in both outbreaks, but while it was once assumed that infected workers would probably show visible cuts, wounds, or lesions on their hands, it was clear in this outbreak that they need not. They had probably transferred the bacteria from their noses.

Some odd but illuminating outbreaks of *S. aureus* have occurred. In 1989 reports of staphylococcal foodborne disease began coming in from several different places. All were traced to canned mush-rooms. In Starkville, Mississippi, 22 people became ill after eating the mushrooms in an omelette and on hamburgers. In Queens, New York, 48 people became ill after sampling the mushrooms in the salad bar. In McKeesport, Pennsylvania, where 12 became ill, it was the mushroom pizza or the parmigiana sauce. In Philipsburg, Pennsylvania, pizza made 20 people ill. In every case staphylococcal enterotoxin was found in samples or in unopened cans of mush-rooms. All the mushrooms were imported from the People's Re-public of China. A recall of these mushrooms was instituted, but not before three other outbreaks were reported. There were only two ways the canned mushrooms could have carried the toxin. They might have had improperly sealed seams, or the *Staphylococcus* grew and produced toxin before the mushrooms were canned. The heat of the canning process destroys bacteria but not toxin, which re-quires longer exposure.

Sometime later the explanation was found. The mushroom-canning facility in China normally obtained its mushrooms from the local area, but as it processed ever greater quantities, they tended to come from farther and farther away. They were brought by farm-ers in plastic bags that allowed them to heat up and produce toxin before canning. This outbreak was truly an anomaly; in the 75 con-firmed staphylococcal outbreaks reported to the CDC's foodborne disease surveillance system between 1982 and 1987, none had been in canned products. But since 50 million pounds of mushrooms were being imported from China each year, the epidemiologists could only wonder what they might have missed.

Staphylococcus aureus

A gram-positive, spherical bacterium (coccus) that looks like a bunch of grapes under a microscope, or sometimes a pair or short chain. Some strains produce a toxin that is resistant to heat and causes illness in humans.

Illness: Staphylococcal food poisoning

Signs and symptoms: Sudden onset of vomiting, cramps, diarrhea, and weakness. There may be headaches, muscle cramping, and increases in blood pressure and pulse rate in severe cases.

Onset time: 2 to 4 hours after eating

Average duration of illness: 2 to 3 days, sometimes longer

Severity: Mild to (rarely) severe

Fatality rate: 0.02

Foods at particular risk of contamination: Meat and poultry dishes; salads made with egg, tuna, chicken, or potatoes; cream-filled baked goods

Nonfood sources: None. Infected humans, animals or equipment can contaminate food where the bacteria produce toxin.

Treatment: The illness is usually self-resolving except in the severely debilitated.

CLOSTRIDIUM BOTULINUM

In September 1996 state and territorial epidemiologists and state public health laboratories got an unusual message from the National Center for Infectious Diseases at the CDC. Italy was in the midst of an outbreak of botulism. It was serious. Seven people had been hospitalized and one had died. The illness, which is characterized by neurological symptoms such as difficulty swallowing, talking, and breathing as well as double vision, can progress to a fatal paralysis of respiratory muscles unless the appropriate antitoxin is given quickly. (The antitoxin is available only from the CDC, which is on duty 24 hours a day to supply it. Physicians who suspect botulism should call their state health department, which will then contact the CDC.) Untreated, 70 percent of those with the infection die.

The Italian cases had been linked to eating several brands of a sweet, soft cheese known as mascarpone. The cheese is used in desserts such as tiramisu, which in the past few years has become increasingly popular in the United States. The problem was a toxin produced by the bacterium *Clostridium botulinum*. It had been found in a number of the cheese samples, and several brands had been recalled and impounded in Italy.

The CDC had gotten its information from the Food and Drug Administration (FDA). Why was it relevant to the state epidemiologists? The cheese had also been exported to the United States where, despite being produced at the same factory in the city of Reggio Emilia, it was being sold under three different names. What happens in Italy—or anywhere else outside the country—is no longer irrelevant to consumers in America. We live in a global food world, and one nation's problems are often now everyone's problems. The FDA quickly checked to see if the implicated lots had reached the United States, found that they had, issued a warning to consumers via the news media, and asked the importer to recall the product, which it did. Of course, recall information often does not reach the public or even shopkeepers, a recent investigation revealed.

There is nothing new about infection with *C. botulinum* toxin. The bacterium is found in soil and can be present on vegetables grown on or in soil, such as potatoes, onions, carrots, and garlic. It prefers an alkaline, low- or no-oxygen environment in which to grow. That is why botulism has long been associated with the consumption of home-canned foods, where the heat of processing is sometimes not enough to kill the spores of the bacteria, which can reproduce in the nonacid, oxygen-free environment of, for example, home-canned green beans. In fact, botulism is a good example of an infection produced when a technique designed to preserve food creates an environment that favors yet another pathogen— something we've been seeing a lot more of recently. A campaign to warn home canners of the problem during the 1940s and 1950s reduced the incidence of botulism in the United States, Canada, and the UK (and probably contributed, along with cultural changes, to the decline of home canning). In recent years outbreaks of botulism have been pretty rare in the United States, although the occasional case from either commercial or home-canned foods still occurs.

The bacterium may also enter the body through wounds and produce a toxin within the body. A case in July 1994 was interesting because both food and an infected wound were initially suspected when an Oklahoman came to the emergency room with the classic symptoms. The patient was admitted to the hospital with dizziness, blurred vision, difficulty swallowing, nausea, and slurred speech. (There are examples of patients who have gone to emergency rooms with these symptoms only to be sent home to "sober up.") Other neurological symptoms, such as facial paralysis, were discovered on examination. When he had trouble breathing, he was put on a respirator. Although the diagnosis was made promptly and he received the botulism antitoxin intravenously, he remained hospitalized for 49 days, 42 of which were on a ventilator. Where had he gotten the infection? He had a wound on his knee, and that might have been an entry point. But during the 24 hours before symptoms had begun, he had eaten a stew containing roast beef and potatoes, and investigators were able to find the toxin in the remaining stew. It had been cooked in a pan with a heavy lid, then left on the stove for three days before being eaten—*without reheating*. Spores had either survived the initial cooking or were introduced afterward. The heavy, tight-fitting lid of the pot had produced the oxygen-free environment that the microbe prefers. Leaving the food out of the refrigerator was what had allowed the bacteria not only to grow but also to produce toxin. While thorough heating will kill bacteria, it takes boiling for 10 minutes to destroy toxin. A similar situation had occurred several years before with commercial pot pies that had not been reheated thoroughly enough to destroy the toxin. But in the case of the stew, even the most basic techniques of safe food handling had been forgotten or ignored.

Some other recent outbreaks have surprised investigators. *C. botulinum* has produced toxin and caused outbreaks in foods that previously wouldn't have been considered risky. It was only as recently as 1983 that researchers discovered that sautéed onions could cause botulism. After three people who had eaten at the same restaurant in Peoria, Illinois, were admitted to the hospital with symptoms of botulism, the health department and the CDC found that onions had been fried in margarine, then kept at the back of the stove to top hamburgers. The sautéing process had not destroyed the botulism spores naturally found on onions, and the margarine had created the anaerobic, or oxygen-free, environment that *C. botulinum* prefers for toxin production.

Another eye-opening outbreak was the result of using chopped garlic packed in oil. The product had been handled carelessly—kept out of the refrigerator for long stretches—and it put 24 patients in the hospital, seven under ventilation. Chopped garlic now has an acid added to prevent *C. botulinum* from growing and producing toxin. Restaurants in the habit of adding garlic to the oil they pour into dishes for bread should be warned to keep it refrigerated, or better yet, to abandon the practice. Flavored oils are now out of favor across the board unless they are commercially prepared with an appropriate acidic additive.

Two other outbreaks of botulism revealed a new potential vehicle but also pointed out how carelessly some restaurants may treat food safety. In both outbreaks potatoes cooked in foil were implicated. Leftover potatoes were not refrigerated and were used in other dishes—in one case, potato salad, and in another, skordalia, a Greek appetizer. Potatoes usually seem clean when they are purchased, so food preparers often don't wash them further, though they may harbor spores of *C. botulinum*. Wrapping and baking the potatoes in foil actually provides a protective layer of steam between potato and skin that prevents the spores from being destroyed. Leaving the wrapped potatoes out at room temperature can create the environment the spores need to produce toxin.

One place where botulism continues to be a significant problem is in Alaska, where investigators identified the source as native foods such as muktuk, a fermented whale dish. Members of many indigenous tribes traditionally prepare fish heads and eggs by letting them ferment in containers buried in the permafrost—or at least that's the way they were once prepared. It was a tradition that prevented the spores of *C. botulinum* from reproducing. Today the dishes aren't prepared as often as they once were, so the preparers have forgotten precisely how to do it. They have opted for plastic buckets and bags as more convenient, and they have often left the food out of the ground to hasten fermentation. The result has been many cases of botulism, a number of them fatal. This is clearly a case of protective traditions being forgotten. The indigenous population has been advised to return to the old ways, which were designed to prevent illness after generations of experience with the process.

There is one other type of botulism. Infants can fall prey to a type all their own. In this case either the living *C. botulinum* or its spores are ingested and then grow in the intestinal tract where the toxin is produced. About 2 percent of infants who get this infection die from respiratory failure. One source of infant botulism is honey, which should never be given to anyone under a year of age because immature digestive systems are less capable of dealing with the bacteria, which apparently present little problem for adults.

A final warning. A previous generation grew up with the information that dented or swollen cans of food were to be avoided. Dents can stress metal and produce microscopic holes that can allow bacteria to enter. Today dented cans regularly appear on grocery store shelves, and the advice to avoid them has seemingly been forgotten. It should be renewed. Swollen cans are an indication that something has gone wrong with the processing, and bacteria have begun to multiply. Never taste food from swollen containers or food that is foamy or has a bad odor. The cause could be *C. botulinum*.

Clostridium botulinum

A member of a group of distinct organisms that are alike only in that they produce similar neurotoxins and are all in the genus *Clostridium*. The organisms are straight to slightly curved, gram-positive (in young cultures), motile, anaerobic rods with oval spores.

Illness: Botulism

Signs and symptoms: Difficulty in swallowing, slurred speech, double vision, difficulty in breathing

Onset time: Usually within 12 to 36 hours of ingesting toxin-containing food

Average duration of illness: Days to months

Severity: Severe

Fatality rate: 65 to 70 percent without treatment, 7.5 percent with treatment

Foods at particular risk of contamination: Non-acidic home-canned foods such as beans, soup mixes, peppers, onions, and potatoes. Sausage, meat, and fish are also susceptible. Tomatoes once had enough acid to make them reliably safe to can at home. This is no longer assured as tomatoes have been bred to be progressively sweeter and may no longer be acidic enough to prevent toxin formation. Extra vinegar can be added during processing to correct this. Commercially canned foods have occasionally been the source of botulism toxin.

Nonfood sources: Open wounds can be exposed to the bacteria, which can then produce toxin that can get into the bloodstream.

Treatment: Antitoxin is available 24 hours a day from the Centers for Disease Control and Prevention. Physicians who suspect botulism should contact their state health department to arrange for shipment of the antitoxin.

CLOSTRIDIUM PERFRINGENS

St. Patrick's Day had come and gone in 1993 when the calls began coming into the Cleveland city health department. The health officers taking them soon noticed the similarity in the victims' stories. All 15 sick individuals had eaten corned beef they had bought from one delicatessen. The local newspaper got wind of the story, and after an article about the outbreak 156 people contacted the department reporting gastrointestinal symptoms within 48 hours of eating food from the deli. Some said they had cramps and vomiting along with the common complaint of diarrhea. Of the 156 people reporting illness, 144 said they had eaten corned beef. When the corned beef was tested, two out of three samples yielded *Clostridium perfringens*. What had gone wrong?

Planning ahead for St. Patrick's Day and what they anticipated would be a big demand for corned beef, the delicatessen had bought 1,400 pounds of raw, salt-cured beef. Several days before the holiday, they had begun boiling portions of the beef, cooling them at room temperature and only then refrigerating them. On March 16 and 17 the portions were put in a warming oven at 120°F before being served. Conclusion: The pieces had been too large to cook thoroughly and cool quickly, and the reheating hadn't been enough to kill the bacteria. In fact, there was just enough heat to encourage it.

That might have been the end of the corned-beef episode, but the story repeated itself just over a week later in Virginia. Again after a belated St. Patrick's Day celebration 86 percent of the 113 people interviewed reported diarrhea, cramps, and sometimes vomiting after eating corned beef. In this case it was a frozen, commercially prepared, brined 10-pound piece of beef that had been cooked in the oven in four batches. Three had been refrigerated, and the last was taken directly to the event. The meat was sliced and put under the heat lamp.

The two outbreaks were not related. The corned beef had been produced by different companies and sold through different distributors. The one thing that linked the two episodes was the insufficient reheating of the corned beef. Heating to an internal temperature of 160°F would have made the meat safe.

The FDA refers to *Clostridium perfringens* as one of the most commonly reported foodborne illnesses in the United States, but most people have never heard of it, and it currently isn't in the top four. However, at least 10 to 20 outbreaks have been reported annually for the past two decades. Outbreaks can result in dozens or even hundreds of sick people because many take place in institutional settings like hospitals, nursing homes, and prisons.

One reason it is so common in institutions is that foods prepared in advance—a typical practice—are sometimes left out and not reheated enough to kill the bacteria that grew happily in the interim. A prison epidemic linked to roast beef, which affected 77 inmates, was followed only a week later by a second traced to ham. (Bad food-handling techniques can be habitual.)

Since the organism is carried in the intestines of infected humans and domestic animals, the spores of the bacteria are often found in the environment in soil or sediment that may be contaminated by animal or human waste. Thus it can find its way into raw foods or onto the hands of food preparers. Infection is likely to occur when a cooked food, which can still contain small numbers of the microbe, is left without refrigeration long enough for the cells to multiply and produce toxin. Gravy that had been prepared and then left out for almost a day before being served was implicated as the source of one outbreak. Ham left too long at room temperature was the troublemaker in another.

C. perfringens food poisoning symptoms, diarrhea and cramps, can begin anywhere from eight to 22 hours after eating a food containing the toxin. Usually it's all over in 24 hours or less, but in some cases milder symptoms can last a week or even two. The few deaths that occur are blamed on dehydration or other complications.

Because the symptoms of *C. perfringens* food poisoning are similar to other foodborne diseases, it can be missed in sporadic cases. The infection is confirmed by looking for the toxin in stool. The bacteria will also be present in the food and in the feces of infected individuals but may be missed in culturing unless a large number of organisms are present.

Clostridium perfringens

A ubiquitous, anaerobic, gram–positive, spore–forming bacillus that frequently contaminates meat and poultry.

Illness: Perfringens food poisoning

Signs and symptoms: Diarrhea, usually with cramps and sometimes vomiting

Onset time: 8 to 16 hours after eating

Average duration of illness: Usually over within 24 hours but can last, rarely, a week or more. (One particular type, rare in the United States, can be very serious and can lead to septicemia, cell and tissue death in the bowel, and death.)

Severity: Usually mild and self–limiting

Fatality rate: Less than 0.1 percent

Foods at particular risk of contamination: Meat, poultry, and seafood dishes

Nonfood sources: None

HEPATITIS A VIRUS

In April 1997 Americans learned through the media of 153 hepatitis A cases in schoolchildren that had been traced to frozen strawberries in school lunches. It might well have been the first they heard of the pathogen. It wasn't that the virus was rare, nor that finding it in frozen strawberries was unique. Two previous outbreaks had, in fact, been traced to frozen strawberries. But for a long time people knew the illness by the name "infectious hepatitis."

Hepatitis A is a member of the same group of viruses, the Picornaviridae family, that includes the common cold and polio viruses. Commonly referred to as HAV, it causes a liver disease, usually mild, characterized by lethargy, fever, nausea, loss of appetite, and after several days, jaundice. Most people recover without long-lasting consequences. The deaths that occur are usually in the elderly, although recent research indicates that people with chronic hepatitis C infections may be at the risk of complete liver failure and death from HAV infection. The CDC estimates that there are 125,000 to 200,000 total HAV infections yearly in the United States with around 100 deaths. However, only 84,000 to 134,000 of these cases may be symptomatic. Thirty-three percent of Americans have evidence of past infection.

What got the attention of the public in the 1997 strawberry outbreak was that it occurred in food distributed to schools, where parents can only hope the food is safe. It is also food that according to USDA regulations is legally required to be produced in the United States, yet the company that distributed the produce had included Mexican berries. This did not mean that the Mexican berries were responsible. Since there were different sources for the berries in the mass-produced product, it was impossible to say precisely where the contamination came from.

Because the infection takes between 10 and 50 days to develop, HAV is only rarely traced to its food source. In those fairly infrequent instances when it has been possible to identify the food through careful epidemiology, the source has run the gamut: cold cuts and sandwiches, fruits and fruit juices, shellfish, salads, milk and milk products, and vegetables. Iced tea and frozen slush drinks have also transmitted the virus.

Often the contamination of food comes from handling by infected workers. Sexual contact with an infected person can also spread the illness. Crowded facilities and poor sanitation make transmission easier.

While HAV could not be called an emerging pathogen, it seems to be a thriving one. A study by the CDC found that reported cases increased 58 percent between 1983 and 1989 alone. It is found worldwide, and often children may not even know they are infected but nevertheless develop immunity. In fact, about 10 percent of people 18 to 19 years of age show immunity; for those over age 50, 65 percent have immunity.

An outbreak that occurred in Oakland County, Michigan, in September 1997 is fairly typical. Of the 37 sick people that health officials interviewed, 33 had eaten at a West Bloomfield delicatessen.

A 67-year-old man died of the infection and five other cases were hospitalized. The source was probably an infected worker; the vehicle was contaminated coleslaw.

About the same time another outbreak started in Washington state. When the running tally of area cases reached 120 by March 1998, the health department took the unusual step of suggesting that people get vaccinated against the infection, because they felt there was a significant risk of more cases appearing.

The vaccine Havrix was licensed for use in the United States in 1995. People advised to get it are those traveling or working in developing countries or in a community with a high level of HAV infection; individuals in high-risk groups, such as intravenous drug users; those engaged in homosexual activity; those with chronic liver disease; and anyone else with a high risk of infection. The vaccine takes about two weeks to become effective. In Seattle many restaurants began seeing that their workers were vaccinated to prevent the contamination of food.

The advice to seek vaccination was controversial. Although the CDC considers the vaccine to be highly effective, the cost of the injection ranges from $40 to $70. With 400,000 people in the area, the community cost might have been as high as $28 million, and the vaccine is of no use after a person has been exposed but before signs of the infection develop. The decision to get vaccinated was left to individuals and their physicians. After exposure, but before infection develops, an injection with immune globulin (IG) can prevent illness. Injections of IG were given to youngsters exposed to the contaminated strawberries during the school lunch outbreak in 1997.

The best way to prevent HAV infection is to avoid contaminated food or drink, but this isn't easy. One thing that may be contributing to the increase of HAV infection is the tendency of people to eat more prepared and raw foods. In December 1996 an outbreak in Los Angeles County was linked to eating foods containing green onions, most of which came from Mexico. There is no guarantee that food preparers are maintaining appropriate hygiene or that they avoid working when ill, and a worker may be infected, and infectious, yet still show no signs of illness. Thus vaccinating food-service workers, as many Seattle restaurants did during the recent outbreak, would help prevent outbreaks from that source. As with most other foodborne pathogens, cooking—or eating cooked foods at restaurants—is the best guarantee. In a rare good-news alert for drinkers, a CDC study found a protective effect against HAV in raw shellfish if, while eating them, you consume beverages with an alcohol content greater than 10 percent—perhaps the original reason for oyster bars. People made logical associations, accurate observations, and drew reasonable conclusions long before there were such things as formal scientific studies.

But the problem of person-to-person transmission through fecal contamination is also growing with social changes. Day-care centers and nursery schools, where youngsters may not be toilet trained or may not wash their hands properly, offer the perfect opportunity for this microbe. Other intimate social settings are equally dangerous. In Australia recently, one boy, already infected—he subsequently came down with symptoms—caused illness in a friend after both bathed in a hot tub. In the summer of 1998 Maricopa County, Arizona, reported the continuing spread of HAV in preschools and day-care centers and began to offer free vaccinations to children ages two to five. The health department began looking into the outbreak a year before, when there was a 40 percent increase in cases from the previous year. More than half the 1998 cases were directly or indirectly linked to day-care contact, a rate that exceeds the national average of 15 percent of cases linked to child care. In a situation such as this, hand washing and other sanitation measures become critical.

Hepatitis A Virus

An enterovirus of the Picornaviridae family.

Illness: Hepatitis

Signs and symptoms: Jaundice, fatigue, abdominal pain, loss of appetite, intermittent nausea, diarrhea

Onset time: 1 to 7 weeks, usually 25 to 30 days from ingestion of the pathogen

Average duration of illness: 1 to 2 weeks usually, extending to months if relapses occur

Severity: Moderate to severe

Fatality rate: 0.3 to 0.4 percent of the reported cases in the United States

Infectious dose: 10 to 100 virus particles

Foods at particular risk of contamination: Shellfish and prepared foods contaminated by infected workers. Foods linked to outbreaks include sandwiches, salads, raw oysters, frozen strawberries, ice and iced drinks, fruits and fruit juices, milk and milk products, and vegetables. Salads, shellfish, and contaminated water are the most common sources.

Nonfood sources: Person-to-person contact with fecal contamination is still the most common means of transmission. Crowded and poor sanitary conditions set the stage, which is why outbreaks are common in prisons, in housing projects, and in the military under adverse conditions. In developing countries, however, outbreaks in adults may be rare because children are often exposed and subsequently develop immunity. During outbreaks day-care workers or attendees may be at risk. Sexual partners of infected individuals and IV drug users are at risk. Individuals at the point of highest infectivity may show no signs of illness.

Treatment: A vaccine is available against hepatitis A, but it must be given well before exposure. There is no treatment, but the illness is self-resolving, although it may be prolonged and relapsing. There is no chronic infection.

NORWALK-LIKE VIRUS

Oysters are eaten virtually around the world. The delicate, fleshy bodies of these mollusks are protected within the satiny lining of their shells. To get at this delicacy, the tightly clamped shells are opened with an oyster knife and the fibrous attachment of oyster to shell is severed. Many people prefer to eat oysters raw, and the only enhancement needed is a squeeze of lemon, a dash of hot sauce, or a dollop of cocktail sauce. Holding the shell in one hand, you can tilt it over your mouth, allowing the oyster to slide in with a minimum of effort. Delicious—and too often today, risky. An oyster filters its environment throughout its system (as do clams, mussels, and other mollusks), and if the water of the bed where the shellfish are growing is not clean, they may pick up, and hold for an extended time, microorganisms that can make diners ill. The culprit may be *Vibrio vulnificus* (see page 93), or it may be a calicivirus called Norwalk-like virus, known in Europe and increasingly around the world as small round-structured virus (SRSV), a practical, descriptive name if ever there was one.

Louisiana is justifiably famous for its oysters, and consuming them is one of the pleasures of visiting the state. But in December 1996 the Louisiana Office of Public Health heard about a cluster of six people who had gotten sick after eating raw oysters at Christmastime. Over the next week or so three more clusters emerged. Everyone who was sick had eaten oysters harvested in Louisiana. Since the state exports its oysters, other states were asked to check if they had cases. Four hundred ninety-three people in 60 clusters were eventually identified as having eaten oysters at gatherings where at least some of the people got sick. The clusters were in Alabama, Florida, Georgia, and Mississippi, as well as Louisiana.

Infection with Norwalk-like virus results in acute gastroenteritis. Characterized by nausea, vomiting, diarrhea, and abdominal cramps, it can be very uncomfortable and is unquestionably inconvenient. But it is usually not terribly serious. Most people recover in a day or two—three at the most—with no apparent long-term or serious health effects.

Caliciviruses, like most viruses, are difficult to detect. The first outbreak associated with these organisms was in Norwalk, Ohio, 30 years ago when schoolchildren became ill with a nonbacterial gastroenteritis. A few years later, with the aid of an electron microscope, the tiny microbe was discovered in their stool samples, and a pathogen was born, or rather, identified. Surely it had been around all along. It is now recognized as an important cause of nonbacterial gastroenteritis. In 1982 an outbreak in Minnesota from contaminated icing on bakery items made 3,000 people ill. The source was a single infected baker who submerged his bare arms into the frosting to mix it—one more reminder of the importance of good hand washing.

Most labs don't have access to the sophisticated molecular methods needed to identify this pathogen. But in ferreting out the culprit in an outbreak, careful interviews can be just as effective as actually finding the virus in the food. What the "ills" who meet the "case definition" have eaten can be compared with what those who have not gotten sick have eaten. If enough of the ills have eaten something that few of the "wells" ate, investigators have most likely identified the "vehicle" in the outbreak.

In the Louisiana outbreak, despite the difficulties of identification, direct electron microscopy revealed SRSVs in some of the fecal samples—and in oysters, which confirmed the findings of the investigation. In attempting to trace the oysters back to their beds, investigators found numerous problems with retail record keeping, which made the investigation more difficult. Sometimes the wholesale records did not match the information on the oyster-sack tags. Outbreaks of this sort often uncover poor record keeping; at the same time, they reveal how important it is to discover what caused the epidemic and, if it is not too late, to get the contaminated food out of the marketplace.

The question was, How had the oysters become contaminated? Only infected human fecal matter transmits SRSVs. When the oysters were traced back to the beds, the investigators looked for an obvious source of raw sewage. It was more difficult to locate than they had imagined. The beds were 12 to 15 miles out to sea and not close to any sewage outlets. It was December, and there were few recreational boats in the area. Could the infection have been transmitted by the oystermen themselves?

It wouldn't be the first time. In 1993, 123 people in Louisiana, Mississippi, Maryland, and North Carolina got sick from eating raw oysters that were also traced to beds off the Louisiana coast. When investigators interviewed fishermen, they discovered that on many of the boats the toilets either flushed directly into the sea or buckets were used as toilets, the contents dumped overboard. The epidemiologists estimated that one infected person, when the waste was dumped overboard, could contaminate an area 100 meters wide and one kilometer long. The oysters were tested repeatedly and found to be contaminated for as long as 25 days after exposure. It was a costly episode for the industry. Oysters that had been shipped to Canada and 17 other states—between 15,000 and 20,000 bushels—had to be destroyed. Harvesting was halted for a week, and although the outbreak was not widely publicized, the reputation of Louisiana oysters wasn't helped among those who did hear about it.

Following the 1993 outbreak, health officials had urged proper holding tanks and waste disposal. That good advice had apparently been ignored; the problem had returned. In fact, the 1996–97 oyster-related outbreak was the third in four years in Louisiana that health officials could attribute to SRSV. Earlier in 1996 an outbreak among workers on an oil rig was traced to a malfunctioning sewage disposal system. Leaks from that sewage apparently resulted in contamination of oyster beds that led to eight clusters of gastroenteritis in four states. Stricter regulation of sewage treatment systems on oil facilities was needed, and in the meantime harvesting oysters from the beds around these sites wasn't a good idea.

What made the 1996–97 outbreak different was that it involved three different beds and three different strains of the virus, suggesting, the investigators thought, that a number of sick oystermen had perhaps vomited or tossed sewage overboard. It seemed perfectly clear to the health investigators, if not to the regulators, that something had to be done about waste disposal on working boats.

Most foodborne pathogens, virtually all in fact, can be cooked out of food. But recently that guarantee has been less certain when the pathogen is Norwalk-like virus. In a recent outbreak some of those made ill had eaten fried oysters and still gotten sick. This is bad news indeed. The question must be, How thoroughly were the fried oysters cooked? But how is someone eating an oyster poor boy in New Orleans supposed to know the answer to that question? It now should be obvious to the shellfish industry that whatever the cost of effective waste disposal on boats, it can't compare to the cost to the industry of another outbreak.

Oysters aren't the only food that can be contaminated with Norwalk-like or small round-structured viruses. A large outbreak occurred among students at Harvard University a few years ago. It was linked to salad that had been contaminated by an infected worker. Once again the importance of thorough hand washing was revealed.

Another suspected outbreak of SRSVs occurred at an elementary school in Dade County, Florida, in October 1996, when 734 of 1,507 students stayed home because of vomiting. The source appeared to be the water, but if it was contaminated, it was a transient occurrence, because no defects were discovered in the supply or the system and the epidemic ended as quickly as it began. Not every outbreak can be solved to everyone's satisfaction. Whatever happened might well happen again—without warning.

Norwalk-like Virus

A family of unclassified small round-structured viruses (SRSVs) that are related to the caliciviruses.

Illness: Infection with SRSV or viral enteritis

Signs and symptoms: Acute gastroenteritis characterized by nausea, vomiting, diarrhea, and abdominal cramps

Average duration of illness: 1 to 3 days

Severity: Mild to moderate

Fatality rate: None

Foods at particular risk of contamination: Shellfish and prepared foods handled by an infected worker; water may be a source.

Nonfood sources: Person-to-person transmission through fecal material

Treatment: None is generally required

CIGUATERA AND OTHER FISH TOXINS

Eden Elieff and her husband, Tom, live just outside of Chicago, where Eden is a teacher and Tom is a dean at the same private secondary school. In June 1996 they were in Jamaica visiting the mother of a student. One day they set out to visit the famous "black sands" of Treasure Beach on the south side of the island. During their three days in the area they had a meal in an offbeat restaurant, run, Eden remembers, by "hippies."

"It was great," says Eden. "There was funky, raw mento music playing. Plenty of steel drums, mandolins, and washboards."

Tom had the chicken, but Eden ordered amberjack, a fish common in Caribbean waters. It wasn't long before her stomach was churning. "I was nauseated, I had fierce runs, but the oddest thing was the sensation of tingling in my arms. Then they began itching frantically. I threw up and felt better, but for 10 days I had low-level nausea and my arms tingled."

She called a local doctor, who professed not to know what was troubling her, and was home before she discovered the cause of her odd symptoms. A friend had been on a Caribbean sailing trip. When he heard that her arms were tingling, he knew at once what the problem was; although he couldn't remember the name, he'd read about the symptoms in a travel guide he'd taken on the trip. Reading it she realized that she'd had a mild case of ciguatera poisoning. If she had read the book before she left, she would have known that the only sure way to avoid exposure to the toxin is to avoid amberjack, barracuda, grouper, mackerel, moray eels, mullet, parrot fish, red snapper, sea bass, and surgeon fish, not only in the Caribbean, but in the South Pacific—in fact, virtually anywhere with coral reefs and warm waters. Fish who graze on certain reefs eat a type of algae that is composed of tiny creatures called dinoflagellates. These organisms produce a toxin that accumulates in the fish. Large fish eat smaller fish, so the bigger the fish, the more toxin it may have accumulated. In fact, smaller sizes of these suspect fish aren't likely to cause trouble.

Unfortunately there is no practical way to test for the toxin in the fish. (It generally requires expensive and complicated bioassay—which is testing a substance against a standard, using an organism such as a mouse—although faster tests are reputedly in the works.) The reaction to it in humans is cumulative. Two people might eat the same fish and only one will become ill because that individual has eaten contaminated fish previously; the toxin has built up in the body to the point of provoking a reaction. Gradually the toxin will clear from both fish and humans, says Robert Dickey, an expert on ciguatera and related toxins with the Food and Drug Administration at the Gulf Coast Seafood Laboratory on Dauphin Island, Alabama.

Eden's illness was typical, although fortunately mild. Symptoms can begin as quickly as 15 minutes after eating or sometimes as late as 24 hours after a meal, but usually they are noticed, as hers were, within several hours of eating a toxin-containing fish. One of the first signs may be a numb feeling to the mouth and tongue, followed by nausea, abdominal pain, vomiting, and diarrhea. The neurological symptoms can vary from mild to life threatening; some people get one symptom but not another. Some are frankly bizarre. In addition to lip and tongue numbness, as well as a painful numbness in the fingers and toes, there can be dental pain and even temperature reversal—cold feels hot. Headache, general weakness, joint and muscle pains, an inability to coordinate movement (ataxia), itching, and even respiratory paralysis and coma also can result. In serious cases the heart can be affected. No definitive test exists to determine if a patient is suffering from ciguatera, but the symptoms are so odd that a clinical diagnosis is fairly easy to make if the physician is alert to the possibility. There is no cure for ciguatera poisoning. Doctors can only support the body and treat the symptoms.

Eden was actually very lucky. While the fatality rate is fairly low at around 1 percent of cases, in some isolated outbreaks up to 10 percent of those poisoned have died, usually from respiratory paralysis or heart failure. Though the symptoms eventually disappear on their own, the tingling and other neurological effects can last for weeks or even months.

Ciguatera poisoning is actually the most common nonbacterial fish-borne poisoning in the United States. Fish both in Florida and from some California waters can be toxic. Since the illness is not reportable, usually only larger outbreaks catch the attention of public health officials, while the numerous sporadic cases such as Eden's that are suspected to occur do not.

In 1991 the Florida Department of Health and Rehabilitative Services heard of eight people who had become ill after eating amberjack in a restaurant. Three people were hospitalized with nausea, vomiting, cramps, diarrhea, and chills and sweats; they then developed itching in their hands and feet along with numbness and muscle weakness. Three more victims turned up. Health officials focused on the fish. The shipment was traced back to a seafood dealer in Key West who had distributed the fish in north Florida through yet another dealer. Part of the lot had been sold to another restaurant in Alabama in addition to the one in Florida, and the rest to a third dealer, who sold the fish to grocery stores in Alabama and north Florida. Reports of more cases surfaced within a few days. Nine people who had bought the fish in the grocery stores became sick. The FDA stepped in and found what it thought were samples of the amberjack from the Key West dealer. Tests found 40 percent to be positive for ciguatera-related biotoxins.

Ciguatera poisonings occur around the world. In January 1998 officials in Hong Kong announced that 50 people had become ill after eating the tiger garoupa fish at a restaurant.

The symptoms of ciguatera poisoning have been recorded in the Caribbean since the 1500s, and the numbers of cases today are thought to be in the tens of thousands in the tropical and subtropical areas of the world. In October 1997 health officials in Hawaii reported 12 ciguatera poisonings after individuals ate kole (surgeon fish) from the north shore of Kauai. Other Hawaiian fish previously linked to the illness are paio, ulua, and roi (grouper).

The question that comes to mind almost at once is, Why is ciguatera causing such a problem on island nations where fish from the surrounding waters have long been a vital and traditional part of the diet? Perhaps the answer is environmental. One source of the toxin is *Gambierdiscus toxicus,* a single-celled dinoflagellate about one-hundredth of an inch in diameter. Other members of the same family have been implicated as well. The distribution of these organisms is uneven in the environment. One side of an island may harbor the creatures, which colonize to produce algae and are frequently found on coral reefs or hard surfaces, such as shipwrecks. They seem to flourish after a major disturbance to a reef, such as a severe storm or dredging or construction on reefs, and some marine biologists question the role of artificially constructed reefs or even dredging or dragging as playing a role in the development of these blooms. While the problem may always have been around, it could well be growing because of environmental changes, since the abundance of the creatures varies with the season, water depth, seafloor conditions, and the temperature and salinity of the water.

Another problem may be that young men have not followed their fathers into professional fishing, where they would learn where and when to fish, but instead have resorted to the occupation when they have needed sudden extra cash, fishing in places their fathers knew to be dangerous. With local fish suspect, the demand for seafood in many of these island nations now far exceeds what is caught locally, which has translated into an increase in imports. Local annual production in the U.S. Virgin Islands is 3.6 million pounds, just over half the 6 million pounds of fish imported. Puerto Rico produces only 15 percent of its domestic needs for seafood. Puerto Rico has, in fact, quarantined sales of the tropical reef-fish species that typically carry ciguatera to reduce the economic consequences resulting from illnesses as well as damage to the fishing industry.

While visitors to the Pacific or Caribbean may be on alert for fish that carry the toxin, diners in some odd places are learning about ciguatera the hard way. In Montreal in November 1996 a menu in a restaurant offered oven-baked barracuda served with vegetables and stewed tomatoes. Five diners became ill on the same day they ate the meal. An alert physician identified the symptoms in two of the five, and the Canadian Center for Disease Prevention and Control investigated, then followed the cases. Three of the five sick individuals first had only gastrointestinal symptoms, one had neurological symptoms, and the remaining patient had both. After six months all the patients were contacted and each had experienced the odd temperature inversion symptom for two to four months. One was still experiencing an itching and burning sensation when the skin was exposed to air. The itching returned after consuming alcohol and cheese. (Other physicians report this as well.)

As the global food trade meets the growing taste for the exotic of consumers everywhere, it's a good bet this restaurant outbreak, in an area where ciguatera wouldn't normally be expected, won't be the last.

Ciguatera isn't the only fish toxin, says Dickey. These "marine biotoxins" as they are called, are the product of harmful algal blooms, such as the massive "red tides," caused by red-tinged dinoflagellates that have multiplied to high concentrations. Dickey explains that in addition to ciguatera, which has a category all its own, the toxins fall into four categories. There is paralytic shellfish poisoning (PSP), caused by a number of species of toxic algae that can contaminate shellfish in the U.S. Northeast and Northwest, as well as other parts of the world; amnesic shellfish poisoning (ASP), found in contaminated mollusks from the U.S. Northeast and Northwest; diarrhetic shellfish poisoning (DSP), found in contaminated shellfish in Japan, southeast Asia, Scandinavia, western Europe, Chile, New Zealand, and eastern Canada; and neurotoxic shellfish poisoning (NSP), which usually results in fish kills and can contaminate shellfish, often along the coast of the Gulf of Mexico and occasionally on the southern Atlantic coast as well as in New Zealand.

Many experts believe that these blooms are spreading and increasing. The number of dinoflagellate species known to be toxic has risen globally from 22 to 55 in recent years.

While outbreaks were once generally noted on the coasts of the United States and Europe, they are now common in Asia and South America—indeed, around the globe. The explanation: Algae species are perhaps being transported in ballast water from ships and encouraged by pollutants that act as nutrients. Unlike the inconspicuous ciguatera blooms, all these toxins are produced by algae with the characteristic red bloom. If you harvest shellfish yourself, it is wise to check with the Coast Guard to see if there are red tides in the area. Regions where there is a red tide will often be posted with warnings, and commercial fishermen track these warnings closely.

They do not monitor the entire ocean, however, and fishermen may unknowingly be at risk. In 1990 eight fishermen on a trip to the Georges Bank 100 miles off Cape Cod, Massachusetts, prepared dinner from mussels incidentally dragged up in their nets. Seven of the crew sat down to eat the feast. Joining them a bit later, the captain, after sampling the mussels, found his crew quickly becoming incapacitated with neurological symptoms. He stayed well just long enough to radio the Coast Guard for help. The fishermen were airlifted to a hospital where they were treated to prevent paralysis of the lungs. All recovered and were back fishing in a few weeks, but the incident might have been tragic if the captain had been on time for his supper.

Scombroid poisoning is from a toxin as well, but it occurs after someone has eaten spoiled fish that have produced a histamine-like substance called saurine. The fish may have a peppery or sharp taste. Flushing of the face, intense headache, nausea and vomiting, and burning and pain in the throat with difficulty swallowing and swelling of the lip may be signs of scombroid toxin ingestion. The symptoms may appear within two hours after eating and should subside within 16 hours. (That's precisely what happened to a surprised group of lawyers in New York City in the summer of 1998 after a fashionable lunch of seared tuna.) Treatment includes getting the material out of the stomach and taking an antihistamine to relieve the distress.

Several other toxins occasionally cause trouble, but they are unlikely to be confronted. Some lamprey eels produce a slime that
seems to contain a toxin that can make people ill, but it is unidentified. The livers and occasionally even the muscle meat of the Green-
land shark have been known to cause severe poisoning. Certain
mullet and goatfish in specific areas at specific times of the year—
the hotter months—contain a toxin that has been linked to central
nervous system symptoms as well as the usual gastrointestinal mani-
festations. Surely the most famous poisoning is that caused by eating
certain parts of the puffer fish called fugu. The mortality rate for
tetrodotoxic poisoning from fugu is 60 percent. Considered a delicacy, this is a fish to avoid unless you have a death wish, although
some Japanese gourmets enjoy the flirtation with danger that comes
from eating it.

Ciguatera and Other Fish Toxins

Fish and shellfish can, after consuming planktonic algae (dinoflagellates, mostly), produce toxins that are poisonous to
humans in various ways.

Illness: Poisoning

Signs and symptoms:

For Ciguatera: Vomiting, diarrhea, neurological symptoms
such as numb mouth and lips, often followed by numbness in
the extremities and itching. There may be a reversal of hot
and cold sensation, dental pain, headache, general weakness,
joint and muscle pains, as well as an inability to coordinate
movement. Severe cases can result in respiratory paralysis,
coma, or heart failure.

PSP: Tingling, burning, or numbness around the mouth,
moving to the face, scalp, and neck, then to the fingertips
and toes. Uncoordinated movements because sensory perception is affected. Dizziness, tightness of the throat and
chest, pain on deep breathing, thirst, and sometimes nausea
and vomiting. A thready and rapid pulse is typical, and super-
ficial reflexes may be absent. If muscular weakness and respiratory distress progress, death may result.

ASP (sometimes called Domoic acid poisoning): Gastrointestinal symptoms followed, in severe cases, by facial

grimace or chewing motion, short-term (in most cases) memory loss, and difficulty breathing.

DSP (no documented cases in the United States): Diarrhea, nausea, vomiting, moderate to severe abdominal pain, and cramps and chills.

NSP: Resembles a mild case of ciguatera or PSP. Tingling of the face that spreads to other parts of the body, cold to hot sensation reversal, dilation of the pupils, and feelings of inebriation. Some victims may experience prolonged diarrhea, nausea, poor coordination, and a burning pain in the rectum.

Onset time:

Ciguatera: From a few minutes to 24 hours after ingesting a toxin-containing fish. Between 2 and 3 hours is average.

PSP: Within 30 minutes of eating

ASP: Between 30 minutes and 6 hours

DSP: Uncertain

NSP: Within 3 hours

Average duration of illness:

Ciguatera: 1 to 4 days for acute illness, with some symptoms possibly lasting as long as several months

PSP: Several days

ASP: Hours to permanent

DSP: Several days

NSP: Several days

Severity:

Ciguatera: Mild to severe

PSP: Mild to severe

ASP: Moderate to severe

DSP: Moderate to severe

NSP: Mild to moderate

Fatality rate:

Ciguatera: 1 to 13 percent

PSP: 1 to 4 percent

ASP: Unknown

DSP: Low

NSP: Low

Foods at particular risk of contamination: In the case of ciguatera, fish that have grazed on coral reefs contaminated by toxin-producing dinoflagellates, especially in the Caribbean or the South Pacific (amberjack, barracuda, grouper, mackerel, moray eels, mullet, parrot fish, red snapper, sea bass, and surgeon fish) or shellfish contaminated by toxin-producing algal blooms, commonly known as red tide; spoiled fish; or fish, such as fugu, that naturally contain toxins. Scombroid toxins are produced in fish that has stayed too long at room temperature.

Nonfood sources: None

Treatment: Supportive as necessary

BACILLUS CEREUS

They were sharing a meal at a Japanese restaurant in Portland, Maine, in September 1985, and the last thing on the minds of this group of friends was getting sick. But before the dinner was even over some were feeling queasy, and then quite suddenly they were nauseated and vomiting, dramatically. They got sicker—the restaurant was pretty much in an uproar—and the health department was called. Because the illnesses had come on so quickly, because it seemed obvious it was something they had eaten there, and because no one could be certain what it was, the owner agreed that the restaurant should be closed immediately. In all, 11 of the 36 people dining that evening vomited or had diarrhea within six hours of eating at the restaurant.

The classic way to approach an outbreak investigation is to determine what each ill individual ate when compared with people who ate in the restaurant but did not become sick. That proved an exercise in frustration because all the patrons had consumed the same items: chicken soup; fried shrimp; stir-fried rice; fried zucchini, onions, and bean sprouts; cucumber, cabbage, and lettuce salad; ginger salad dressing; hibachi chicken and steak; and tea. As is often the case in Japanese or Chinese restaurants, most people tried each other's dishes. The result: food confusion, an epidemiologist's worst nightmare. But the health department had some success. Samples from the sick individuals cultured an organism called *Bacillus cereus*. It was also found on the hibachi steak.

It would seem fairly obvious that the steak was the cause, but Dr.

Kathleen Gensheimer of the Maine Bureau of Health wasn't satis-
fied. The meat was a very unlikely source of the bacteria and it
could have been contaminated by another food. What seemed a
more likely vehicle was the fried rice, customarily made from leftover boiled rice. The restaurant staff wasn't quite sure whether it had
been refrigerated or stored at room temperature. Nothing could
ever be proved, but there were any number of good, solid reasons to
suspect rice.

B. cereus, as its name implies (Ceres was a Roman goddess of
agriculture, and it is from her that we get the word cereal), is often
found on rice. The bacteria are ubiquitous in the environment.
B. cereus spores have been found on cereals, beans, vegetables, spices,
and powdered and fresh milk. When the bacterium germinates, it
produces a toxin that can cause food poisoning. A common source
of the toxin is cooked food that has been left out at room temperature, then reheated.

The suddenness of the illness was a clue. B. cereus actually causes
two different sets of symptoms. One is a diarrheal malady not unlike
that produced by infection with Clostridium perfringens. It can take
between 10 and 12 hours to manifest itself after someone eats contaminated food and is caused by a heat-labile toxin produced by the
bacteria. The other is caused by a heat-stable toxin from B. cereus
and is characterized by a rapid onset of dramatic vomiting. Someone who has eaten contaminated food can show signs of illness as
soon as an hour after eating. The average is between one and six
hours. This last symptom—vomiting is properly called an emetic
syndrome—has almost always been associated with fried rice from
restaurants serving Oriental dishes since it is a normal practice to
boil large quantities of the grain. The problem arises when the rice
is set aside without refrigeration.

Numerous outbreaks of B. cereus have been traced to fried rice,
and caterers and restaurants have received many warnings about
keeping rice at room temperature. But the outbreaks continue.

In 1993 at two jointly owned day-care centers in northern Virginia, some of the staff and children became violently ill after eating
a catered lunch. The symptoms included various combinations of
nausea, abdominal cramps, and diarrhea. Some became sick quite
quickly; the median incubation period was two hours. But the ill-

ness passed just as quickly. Within approximately four hours they were pretty well over it.

Fried rice prepared at a local restaurant was quickly implicated. It had been cooked the night before and cooled at room temperature before being refrigerated. The next morning it was fried in oil with cooked chicken and taken to the centers. It was never refrigerated at the day-care center and was served without reheating. Apparently educating restaurant workers is an ongoing challenge.

To avoid this problem, the rice must be refrigerated promptly, (below 41°F or 5°C) then reheated thoroughly (above 140°F or 60°C).

Bacillus cereus

A common, spore-forming, aerobic, gram-positive rod that is found throughout the environment.

Illness: *B. cereus* food poisoning, either diarrheal or emetic (vomiting).

Signs and symptoms: Causes two different sets of symptoms depending on the toxin: (a) a diarrheal malady similar to that caused by *Clostridium perfringens* food poisoning; (b) an emetic syndrome (vomiting) with occasional diarrhea and/or cramps

Onset time: (a) average incubation period of 10 to 12 hours; (b) average incubation period 0.5 to 6 hours

Average duration of illness: (a) 1 to 2 days; (b) less than 24 hours

Severity: (a) mild to moderate; (b) violent but short-lived

Fatality rate: None

Foods at particular risk of contamination: The diarrheal malady (a) has been linked to meats, milk, vegetables, and fish. The emetic syndrome (b) is usually linked to rice products, but other starchy foods have been implicated; sauces, puddings, soups, casseroles, and salads have also been associated with outbreaks.

Nonfood sources: None

Treatment: None usually required; rehydration in serious cases.

THE VIBRIOS

In July 1997 a Spanish-speaking construction worker in Maracopa County, Arizona, stopped by a street market to pick up fresh shrimp as a treat. He liked them, as many people do, soaked in lemon or lime juice, which turns raw seafood into a dish called seviche. It's thought that the soaking in the acidic lemon or lime is a kind of chemical "cooking" or pickling process that will kill any pathogens that might be lurking about (although public health officials frown upon the practice, since no tests have been done to prove its effectiveness). But instead of soaking the shrimp, the adventurous and trusting diner merely squeezed lemon juice on them and popped them into his mouth.

A day or so later he began feeling ill with nausea, vomiting, cramps, and unrelenting watery diarrhea—at least 25 episodes a day. It was serious enough to send him to the hospital, where he was rehydrated in the emergency room. A stool culture revealed something the hospital did not expect to see. The patient was suffering from cholera. The hospital notified the county's public health department at once.

Cholera is a disease of someplace else. Caused by the bacterium *Vibrio cholerae,* a rod-shaped bacterium with a commalike shape, and spread by fecally contaminated water, cholera is something we think of as happening in underdeveloped countries where sanitation and water and sewage treatment may be poor. It was cholera that caused the deaths of 33,000 Rwandan refugees in 1994 in Zaire when more than 100,000 helpless and homeless people were dependent on a contaminated water supply. It can be a frightening disease because the copious amounts of watery diarrhea produces rapid and extensive dehydration that, without treatment, can kill within a matter of hours. Yet the treatment, in the early stages of the infection, can be simple. A solution made from an inexpensive mixture of sodium chloride, sodium bicarbonate, potassium chloride, and dextrose can be administered spoonful by spoonful, and miraculously the oral rehydration solution, as it is called, can save lives by preventing the potentially fatal dehydration and electrolyte imbalance.

Prior to 1991 there had been no epidemic of cholera in the Americas for over a century, but in that year cases began to break out in Peru from a strain, *Vibrio cholerae* O1 biotype El Tor, that since 1961 had been causing a relentlessly spreading pandemic in Africa and Oceania. In the Americas it now has, in less than a decade, made more than a million people seriously ill and killed more than 10,000 in an epidemic that is not over. Cases in the United States have increased accordingly, not from the water supply, which is generally clean, but from international travelers or contaminated food that has found its way into the country. In 1992, 102 cases of cholera were reported in the United States—three times as many as in any year since 1961, when the Centers for Disease Control and Prevention (CDC) began keeping records. Some individuals have gotten sick from crabs or other foods their relatives brought into the country from Central America. A widespread outbreak in the United States occurred after a plane trip from South America on which seafood salad was served. One of the 75 sick passengers died. Several people in Maryland got cholera, although an Asian strain, from contaminated frozen coconut juice from Thailand, demonstrating how easy it is for the global food trade to move the bacillus around the world.

The CDC identified the strain in the Arizona man as the one spreading its misery through South and Central America, and the Arizona Department of Health Services subsequently detected other cholera strains on shrimp from the market. Tracking the shrimp proved almost impossible, but 360 pounds of it, some thought to be from Ecuador, were embargoed by the Maricopa County Environmental Services Department.

Actually, we have our own strain of *Vibrio cholerae* in the United States, which happens to be one of only two places in the world where the bacillus has settled happily into the ecosystem—in this case, the Gulf Coast—and become endemic. Fortunately it is the type, called non-O1, that does not seem to cause widespread outbreaks or dangerous disease, but it does cause sporadic cases of home-grown if milder cholera among those who eat raw or less than thoroughly cooked shellfish, especially crabs and oysters, harvested from the area.

A nasty cousin of *V. cholerae* named *Vibrio vulnificus* also seems fond of the warm Gulf waters, causing more and more illnesses recently and reaching the status of being viewed as an emerging foodborne pathogen. It is the most vicious of the foodborne pathogens, killing 50 percent of the people it infects. The illness is characterized by gastroenteritis in healthy people, but in people with underlying chronic diseases, the microorganism can enter the bloodstream and produce septicemia or septic shock, which can rapidly be followed by death. About 70 percent of these cases have characteristic bulbous skin eruptions as well. (*V. vulnificus* can also affect the skin directly when people with open wounds bathe in contaminated water or are exposed to the drippings from seafood. About 25 percent of these infections are fatal.) Those most vulnerable to *V. vulnificus* are those with chronic liver disease or compromised immune systems, whether from cancer treatments or some other cause such as excessive alcohol consumption.

There are probably a number of reasons for the recent increase in cases. More individuals have compromised immune systems, for one thing: more people undergoing challenging cancer therapies or receiving organ transplants, more individuals with AIDS. *Vibrio vulnificus* is thought to be a natural inhabitant of the oceans, but the growing pollution of our offshore waters may be giving this pathogen a lot of encouragement.

Last but not least, people almost universally have discarded or ignore Mother's famous dictum to eat raw shellfish only in months with an *R*. This admonition has nothing to do with some magical quality to that particular letter but to the fact that sea waters are cooler in these *R*, or winter, months and thus less encouraging to the growth of *V. vulnificus*. Virtually all the cases of infection with the pathogen occur in the summer; in fact, the bacillus has been found in up to 50 percent of the oyster beds in the Gulf of Mexico during warm months (at least in the Northern Hemisphere). And sometimes the illnesses occur far from where the oysters (implicated in more than 96 percent of infections) are harvested. In the Los Angeles area in 1996 during the *R*-less month of May, three deaths were linked to eating raw oysters from Galveston Bay in Texas and Eloi Bay, Louisiana.

There are other members of the *Vibrio* genus that can cause trouble. Infection with *Vibrio parahaemolyticus* has been associated with diarrhea, abdominal cramps, nausea, vomiting, headache, fever, and chills. The illness tends to be on the mild to moderate side, but serious cases may need hospitalization. A vast outbreak in 1998 that made 368 people ill in seven states was linked to oysters from Galveston Bay. After an investigation it was found that the source of the *V. parahaemolyticus* was probably a ship discharging ballast water. This outbreak was the largest one yet for shellfish.

Other *Vibrio* serotypes have also been associated with diarrheal disease. That is, they have been found in cultures taken from patients when no other pathogens could be found, but the link is not conclusive.

The surest way to avoid infection with *Vibrio cholerae* is to avoid contaminated drinking water and any foods contaminated water might have touched. In areas where cholera is present, cooking foods thoroughly and eating them while they are hot, together with drinking only bottled, carbonated, or boiled water, is a sound strategy. Does avoiding the other Vibrios mean giving up raw shellfish entirely? The identification of Gulf oysters as a risk factor for contracting these illnesses has been hard on the shellfish industry there. In fact, relative to the large numbers of oysters sold and eaten, the infection rate is fairly small. Nevertheless, given the potential deadly seriousness of the infection for those with chronic liver disease or an impaired immune system, the only reasonable course is for these individuals to avoid all raw or undercooked shellfish. Others might want to weigh their risks carefully, remembering that shellfish are not only safe if thoroughly cooked, they can be delicious as well.

The Vibrios

A bacillus with a curved, commalike shape, typically found in water. Disease is caused by the cholera strains when the organism attaches itself to the small intestine of infected individuals. *V. cholerae* produces a toxin that is an invasive mechanism, and the action of a toxin is suspected but not identified in *V. parahaemolyticus*.

Illness: *V. cholerae:* Cholera; *V. parahaemolyticus:* infection with *V. parahaemolyticus; V. vulnificus:* infection with *V. vulnificus*

Signs and symptoms: Different members of this group have different patterns of disease.

V. cholerae O1: Symptoms may vary from a mild, watery diarrhea to an acute diarrhea, with characteristic rice-water stools that occur along with abdominal cramps, nausea, vomiting, dehydration, and shock. Death can occur after severe fluid and electrolyte loss.

V. cholerae non-O1: Milder diarrhea with abdominal cramps, and fever. Nausea and vomiting occur in some people. About 25 percent of patients will have blood and mucus in their stools.

V. parahaemolyticus: Diarrhea, abdominal cramps, nausea, vomiting, headache, fever, and chills. The illness is usually mild or moderate, although some cases may require hospitalization.

V. vulnificus: Gastroenteritis with cramps, nausea, vomiting

Onset time:

V. cholerae O1: May have a sudden onset; incubation varies from 6 hours to 5 days.

V. cholerae non-O1: Diarrhea usually occurs within 48 hours of ingestion but 3 days is possible.

V. parahaemolyticus: Symptoms can begin between 4 and 96 hours after eating, but 15 hours is about average.

V vulnificus: Symptoms usually occur within 16 hours of ingestion.

Average duration of illness:

V. cholerae non-O1 and O1: Diarrhea may last 6 to 7 days and may be severe.

V. parahaemolyticus: Usually mild, the illness may last only 2 to 3 days.

V. vulnificus: Varies from brief to lengthy according to the health status of the infected person.

Severity:

V. cholerae O1: May be severe

V. cholerae non-O1: Mild to moderate

V. parahaemolyticus: Usually mild to moderate and self-limiting

V. vulnificus: Varies greatly from mild to deadly according to the health status of the individual infected

Fatality rate:

V. cholerae O1: Variable according to conditions. In the United States it is 1 percent or less.

V. cholerae non-O1: Greater than 1 percent

V. parahaemolyticus: Greater than 1 percent

V. vulnificus: 0–50 percent in immune–compromised individuals when the infection enters the bloodstream

Foods at particular risk of contamination:

V. cholerae O1: Contaminated water and anything it touches, such as vegetables, have spread the disease among communities in South America that do not have modern water facilities. Ballast water from ships has contaminated U.S. waters. Sporadic cases have occurred from imported foods or from airplane meals.

V. cholerae non-O1: Shellfish harvested from U.S. coastal waters, particularly the Gulf of Mexico. Eating raw, improperly cooked, or cooked and recontaminated shellfish from these waters may lead to infection.

V. parahaemolyticus: Raw, improperly cooked, or cooked and recontaminated fish and shellfish have been linked to outbreaks. More infections occur in the warmer months of the year.

V. vulnificus: Oysters, clams, and crabs. Consumption of these products raw or recontaminated may result in illness.

Treatment:

V. cholerae O1: Rehydration

V. cholerae Non-O1: Antibiotics such as tetracycline can shorten the severity and duration of the illness.

V. parahaemolyticus: usually self-limiting; hospitalization in rare cases.

V. vulnificus: supportive (Primary septicemia, a life-threatening condition requiring hospitalization, may occur in individuals with diabetes, cirrhosis, leukemia, or who take immunosuppressive drugs or steroids.)

YERSINIA

There is nothing really new about *Yersinia enterocolitica*. The pathogen has been around a long time and is found in animals and in the environment. It was linked to human illness, however, only in the 1960s. What is new is that infection with the pathogen is appearing ever more frequently around the world. In 1976 the World Health Organization described the spread of this bacterium as "dramatic" and "impressive," both in animals and in humans, and in 1995 declared it one of the important emerging foodborne pathogens. Several factors may be responsible, including the increasing intensive rearing of pigs. In fact, the rise in *Yersinia* infections has precisely paralleled the movement in developing countries to raise pigs in factory-like conditions. The large numbers, the close quarters, the various stresses the animals experience, and the lack of diversity in the herds are factors that encourage the spread of any pathogenic organism in food animals.

Since *Yersinia* is often found in pigs, it shows up as a human disease most frequently among pork eaters, especially those individuals who prepare dishes that require a great deal of handling, or those who have the bad habit of nibbling at raw sausage. Thus the countries where people eat more pork, such as in northern Europe and the Far East, have more cases of infection with this pathogen.

The microbe has the unfortunate habit of growing nicely at refrigerator temperature. It is one of those pathogens that make one think that for every two steps forward in food safety, we collectively take one step backward.

Yersiniosis is the name of the ailment caused by this bacterium. It is characterized by fever and abdominal pain that may include vomiting and diarrhea. The symptoms are often mistaken for appendicitis, and unnecessary surgeries are not uncommon.

A few years ago the CDC noticed an increase in yersiniosis in Atlanta, its own backyard so to speak. When its epidemiologists investigated the cases—mainly in young children—they found that a risk factor for infection in a child was an African-American mother preparing chitterlings. Preparing this traditionally seasonal dish out of pig intestines is a time-consuming and hands-on task. It now appears that since the intestines may harbor *Yersinia,* the task may be a

dangerous one, not only for the preparer but for children playing in
the kitchen while the preparation is under way. The bacterium can
be passed from person to person on hands or whatever the intestines touch.

A subsequent education campaign on the safe preparation of
this dish was apparently successful. There hasn't been another
chitterling-associated outbreak. Of course, it may also be that people have just abandoned the dish, which is a shame, as it represents
yet another loss of cultural expression and a food tradition.

Outbreaks of yersiniosis are infrequent in the United States, and
two of the most recent were not directly linked to pigs, although in
one a pig wallowed in the background. In 1995 the Vermont State
Health Department was notified by a medical center in nearby
New Hampshire that three Vermont residents had tested positive for
Y. enterocolitica. Within a week or so two more cases were reported,
one a Vermont resident and the other from New Hampshire. Eventually there would be 10 cases of yersiniosis. They were not mild
cases. Three patients were hospitalized, and one underwent an unnecessary appendectomy.

The link between the cases turned out to be a particular dairy
that sold pasteurized milk. The facility seemed clean and sanitary
and the process without defect. Milk samples were also clean. The
only possible means of transmission seemed to be that the farm also
kept pigs, and the employee who cared for the pigs also handled
both empty and filled milk bottles. *Y. enterocolitica* was found in one
of the pigs, but it was a different strain from that found in the patients. Of course some time had elapsed between the illnesses and
the testing of the pig. The health department feels certain they discovered the cause of the illnesses and the source of the bacterium;
the dairy owner, not surprisingly, disagrees. Sometimes outbreaks
can be easy to solve; other times they are impossible. *Yersinia* seems
particularly frustrating.

That was definitely the case in Texas in the summer of 1997. In
June the laboratory at the Texas Department of Health reported five
cultures positive for *Y. enterocolitica*. The report immediately got the
attention of the department's Infectious Disease Epidemiology and
Surveillance Division. The health department seldom saw *Yersinia*
cases, and these had something in common. They were all infants—

most less than a year old. They'd been cultured because they all had
bloody diarrhea.

The division sent out a fax alert at once to acute-care facilities
across the state asking physicians to be on the lookout for other
cases, and before long reports began coming in. Clearly the state was
in the midst of an outbreak. David Bergmire-Sweat, an epidemiologist in the division, organized an investigation along typical lines.
Once questionnaires were developed and a suitable control group
set up, the interviews began. They were long questionnaires, but
they turned up no single food or activity common to either the infants or the families. It was frustrating, and team members went
back and did more interviews with families while looking for more
cases throughout the state. "We tried harder on this than any cluster
I've ever investigated," Bergmier-Sweat recalls.

But the outbreak was a tease. Nothing was statistically significant.
There *was* one tantalizing clue. No breast-fed infants were among
the 11 strongest cases and suspects (nine culture-confirmed cases
and two very sick babies with bloody diarrhea). A single contaminated batch of formula might be the cause, they speculated, but
proving it would be difficult.

Bergmire-Sweat goes over all the reasons the culprit was so elu-
sive. "It took several days for the disease to incubate," he says,
"maybe another day or two for the child to be taken to the physician."

Then the doctor might have suspected *Shigella,* which is self-
resolving, and not ordered a culture. Or if a culture was taken, the
local lab might not have looked for *Yersinia* anyway, since it requires
a special culture medium. *Yersinia* was not then on the list of reportable infectious diseases in Texas, so even if it were found, the
health department wouldn't have been notified. Even with cases
that appeared after the alert, the process took time. It was a few days
before Bergmire-Sweat was able to reach a family.

"If it was infant formula, what we tested at that point probably
wouldn't have been what the child was drinking when he got sick.
There was no association with any one brand, but then people
change brands," he says. Bergmire-Sweat checked with the CDC to
see if other states were reporting an increase in cases of yersiniosis,
but none were. Of course, he says, this might simply have been be-

cause most labs don't routinely culture for the pathogen. "By September we had no more cases. All we know now is that for two
months in the summer of 1997 in Texas we had an outbreak of
yersiniosis that affected more than 20 infants. Many of them were
seriously ill, and some of them required hospitalization. Nine cases
had positive cultures for *Y. entercolitica* and others were suspicious.
The cases were scattered around the state, not clustered. They were
all formula fed, but there was no association with any brand. When
all was said and done, we couldn't prove anything."

The Texas Department of Health had spotted an outbreak, but
no one will ever know the cause or how such an outbreak might be
avoided in the future. Bergmire-Sweat is dogged by the frustrating
memory. "I think if it had been possible to find the cause, I would
have." The scattered nature of the cases leads one to think that it
might have been from a mass-produced and widely distributed food
product, and formula seemed obvious, but it is the nature of outbreaks from such foods that they elude detection. Only because the
Texas state lab routinely cultured for *Yersinia* was it spotted at all.
Because *Yersinia* wasn't a reportable pathogen, Bergmire-Sweat
didn't know if what they were seeing was way out of line or not.
He just knew they'd never seen it before.

Infection with *Yersinia* is now reportable in the state, so if more
cases appear, epidemiologists will be able to check back to see if the
number is out of the ordinary. Finding it in Texas was a confirma-
tion of the fact that you find what you are looking for. It could also
mean that, because so few labs test regularly for the pathogen, sporadic cases and even outbreaks are being missed.

Two other species of the *Yersinia* genus cause illness in humans.
Y. pseudotuberculosis has been transmitted by food and water in Japan,
but has so far caused no trouble in the United States. The wicked
cousin of the genus is *Y. pestis,* which cases plague, and although
there is a reservoir of this pathogen in the American West, it is not
transmitted via food.

Yersinia

Yersinia enterocolitica, a small, rod-shaped, gram-negative bacterium.
Illness: Yersiniosis

Signs and symptoms: Fever and abdominal pain, similar to appendicitis or mesenteric lymphadenitis, along with gastrointestinal symptoms of diarrhea and vomiting. It can be misdiagnosed as appendicitis or Crohn's disease. The bacteria can also cause infection in joints, wounds, and the urinary tract.

Onset time: Usually between 24 and 48 hours after ingestion of the organism

Average duration of illness: Days to weeks

Severity: Mild to moderate, self-limiting

Fatality rate: 0.03 percent

Foods at particular risk of contamination: Outbreaks have been linked to pork, and strains of *Y. enterocolitica* can be found in other meats, oysters, fish, and raw milk. An outbreak was linked to pasteurized milk, and another in infants appeared to be caused by formula, but the source remained unproven.

Nonfood sources: None

Treatment: Supportive

WATERBUGS

CRYPTOSPORIDIUM PARVUM

It's fair to say that before the spring of 1993 most Americans had never heard of *Cryptosporidium parvum* or given any thought at all to what this parasite might mean to their lives. It isn't that the pathogen hadn't been around—it had been—but it was on April 5 of that year that health officials in Milwaukee, Wisconsin, began noticing something was amiss in their city. Drug stores were running out of diarrhea medicine, and an unusual number of people were reporting what the local newspaper, perhaps for lack of a better word, would call "flulike" symptoms. At first public health officials suspected they might be in the midst of some sort of viral epidemic. (This seems always to be the first thought among public health officials, although the viral causes of foodborne disease remain in fifth place in the order of cases caused.) Throughout the city there was widespread absenteeism at schools, among teachers and students, and among hospital employees. The tests that had been done on some of the victims were inconclusive until April 7, when *Cryptosporidium* oocysts, or egglike forms, were identified in two of seven stool samples. Since labs had come up with nothing else, public health officials thought they had the villain. The logical source was the water supply; no other single food or drink was likely to have reached so many people, and "crypto," as it is known, is often found in water. The records of the two water plants were hurriedly checked, and the operators found an increase in turbidity, a kind of cloudiness that usually spells trouble. It had begun around March 21, then spiked to unprecedented levels between March 23 and April 5. On April 7, Milwaukee's mayor, John Norquist, advised city residents to boil their water before drinking it or washing food in it. The city's water was chlorinated, but chlorine didn't kill this bug, at least not in the amounts acceptable in drinking water. (Fortunately for Milwaukee, a city with a brewing tradition, they had beer, which some hotels were telling worried tourists was "Milwaukee's version of bottled water.")

More than 800,000 people in the area get their drinking water from the South Milwaukee waterworks plant. When the numbers of ill were finally tallied and the extent of the outbreak estimated months later, more than 400,000 people—over half of those using that supply—had probably been infected. The causes were complex, but possible contamination from cattle waste, flooding, and human error were all implicated. It was the largest waterborne outbreak ever reported in the United States, and for Americans, who had long considered their water the best and safest in the world, it was a rude awakening to the thought that what comes out of the tap might not be safe after all.

Among the ill was Julie Drews, a teenager with cancer who had been undergoing chemotherapy at a Milwaukee hospital. Infected with the parasite from the city's water, she had continuous and unrelenting diarrhea that was often bloody. Her weight plummeted, she weakened to the point that she had to be carried, and she would double over from the waves of intense stomach pain, her mother told reporters. There was no effective medical treatment for the infestation. A healthy person can usually fight off infection, but Julie's immune system, impaired by the cancer treatments, could not cope. She died in October, six months after the initial infection, at the age of 17. More than 100 deaths were linked to infection with the microbe. Most were among AIDS patients, for whom infection is potentially deadly, but anyone with a damaged immune system is at particular risk.

Cryptosporidium parvum is called an emerging pathogen because it was so seldom seen in the past and not thought to cause human illness until recently. Suggestions are that it is also being newly spread in the environment for a variety of reasons, some related to changes in lifestyle, social organization, and agriculture. Today experts such as Dr. Richard L. Guerrant of the University of Virginia School of Medicine consider it a major threat to the U.S. water supply. As if to make that point, eight months after the Milwaukee outbreak residents of Washington, D.C., awoke to their own crypto-initiated, boil-water alert. The Pentagon's 600-plus water fountains were turned off, and bottled water was the order of the day in offices across the city. Stores quickly ran out of supplies. It was particularly unsettling to find the nation's capital so vulnerable, but any city that doesn't filter its water to a high standard is at risk. In fact, many water-related outbreaks of cryptosporidiosis, as the illness is known, have been verified in the United States. One study found the oocysts present in 27 percent of the 66 drinking-water samples taken in 14 states.

Like many human pathogens, *Cryptosporidium* was first recognized by veterinarians. The parasitic protozoan, about one-hundredth the size of a speck of dust, was linked to human disease only in 1976, and between 1976 and 1982 only seven cases were reported in humans. Five of these were in immune-suppressed individuals, and the increase in infection has paralleled the increase in AIDS. *C. parvum* does not grow in food, but the oocysts can survive in wet, moist foods that have been contaminated. The parasite can be transmitted by fecally contaminated water (not just drinking water but swimming and wading pools), contaminated foods, infected animals, and direct person-to-person contact.

Today *Cryptosporidium* is recognized as a cause of severe, often irreversible and life-threatening diarrhea in patients with AIDS. In one study their fatality rate was 55 percent. But crypto can also

cause debilitating diarrhea in previously healthy individuals, and as
the Milwaukee outbreak demonstrated, a large outbreak can have a
profound economic impact on a community, as everything from
commerce to tourism to health care is affected.

The *Cryptosporidium* oocysts need a host to reproduce. Infection
can take place with as few as 30 microscopic oocysts, and it takes
between two and 10 days following ingestion for the oocysts to incubate. The tiny critter attaches to the wall of the intestine and re-
produces in a complex cycle. In a healthy person the illness can last
as long as two weeks, sometimes less, but a person can begin to recover and then become ill again. The first tests for crypto were invasive, but faster, more efficient, and cheaper laboratory tests are
now widely available. They still may be relatively expensive, and
they may not always be sensitive enough to spot the microbes unless
the organisms are plentiful in the stool.

There is no approved or standard treatment for the infection except to supportively treat the typical symptoms: profuse watery diarrhea, painful abdominal cramping, weight loss (the average weight
loss in one outbreak was 10 pounds), vomiting, and low-grade fever.
Oral rehydration solution can be taken to stave off dehydration. Antibiotics aren't considered effective, although one antibiotic has been
found in studies to be useful in reducing the *amount* of diarrhea in
AIDS patients. When the infection becomes chronic, as it does in
many of the severely immune-compromised, other organs can become infected.

The mature oocysts are excreted in the feces, sometimes by individuals who show no sign of infection, and contact with infected
fecal material is the source of secondary, person-to-person infection. Day-care facilities, nursing homes, and hospitals are vulnerable
to person-to-person transmission, and a high degree of hygiene and
frequent hand washing is advisable in these settings, as in any situation where there is fecal contact. Fourteen outbreaks have been
documented in the United States in day-care centers. As is always
the case, contact with human and animal waste needs to be avoided,
and all fecal material must be managed in a manner that doesn't
contaminate anything people ingest or put into their mouths.

Although *Cryptosporidium* is most frequently found in water,
outbreaks from foods have occurred. In 1993 in Maine the state

epidemiologist learned that many of the students—too many—at several schools in one area were absent because of gastrointestinal symptoms. The 230 that were ill, it was quickly determined, had attended an agricultural fair organized by high school students. A few days after the first reports, *Cryptosporidium* was found in the stools of three of the ill. A study using a questionnaire soon linked the illnesses to freshly pressed cider at the fair. The two investigators, State Epidemiologist Dr. Kathleen Gensheimer, and her assistant, Dr. Peter Mallard, on assignment to the state while undergoing CDC training for the Epidemic Intelligence Service (EIS), were able to piece together the story of how the cider became contaminated. They were even able to find the pathogen in the cider itself when they discovered that a student had taken a bottle home (for the purpose of hardening it, or turning it into an alcoholic beverage, an age-old country tradition). The five bushels of apples used in the morning had been bought from a commercial orchard, but when the students making the cider ran out of apples at midday, they resorted to gathering more apples from old trees on the edge of a pasture where cows had recently grazed. Oocysts of *Cryptosporidium* were found in a calf that had been grazing in the pasture; they were also found on the press. Although the apples had been washed, it was not thorough enough to prevent spreading the oocysts throughout the juice during the pressing. Sadly, freshly made apple cider and other fresh, unpasteurized juices are now known to be risk factors for infection with pathogenic organisms. Many juice producers have responded by using a "flash" pasteurization for the apple juice in their otherwise fresh products. It is said to retain the fresh flavor without the pathogens.

More recently, in December 1997 a number of people began getting sick in Spokane, Washington. What they had in common was a banquet at a local restaurant a week earlier. It was a while before public health officials suspected crypto, but the long incubation period between the illnesses and the banquet led them to suspect a parasite. Eight of 10 stool specimens from the ill were positive for *Cryptosporidium*. Since there had been 18 separate food and beverage items—seven of them uncooked—at the banquet, it wasn't easy sorting out what was responsible. No single food stood out, but when the investigators looked at foods that contained green onions, 51 of the sick people could recall having eaten them. It was never entirely clear what had happened, but there were clues. The green onions were never washed before being cut up and used in dishes. Two of the food-service workers were also positive for crypto infection, one symptomatic and one asymptomatic. Another remembered being sick during December. But all had also eaten the banquet foods associated with the outbreak.

Twenty years ago one worried about the safety of water abroad; it's fair to say that more and more people are now worried about the safety of water here at home. While infection for a healthy person can be no more than a severe nuisance, a widespread outbreak can entirely disrupt a community, and anyone who is immunocompromised needs to be absolutely vigilant about avoiding water contaminated with this microorganism. How does one do that? The CDC has suggested that those with compromised or less well developed immune systems consult their physicians before drinking tap water. The American Water Works Association recently went still further, warning HIV-infected individuals to boil their tap water before drinking it. Bringing it to a roiling boil for one minute is sufficient. It should then cool naturally. Don't add ice, which may be contaminated.

Bottled water may or may not be safe, as proper filtration is the answer to avoiding *Cryptosporidium*. (It should be noted that surface water from reservoirs is the problem. Groundwater drawn from deep underground supplies that has not been recontaminated during bottling will not harbor these parasites.) Those needing to pay special attention to water quality should make certain that bottled water is labeled with one or more of the following before it is considered safe: "reverse osmosis," "tested and certified by NSF Standard 53 for cyst reduction," or "absolute micron size of one micron or smaller." Any of these guarantee the removal of *Cryptosporidium*. If the information is not on the bottle, call the company's toll-free number and ask. If it is properly filtered, ask to have that information and a complete analysis of the water sent to you. Any home filtration system relied on by the immunocompromised should meet the same standard, and the filter should be changed according to instructions *by a healthy individual,* as it may be contaminated. Other maintenance procedures should be carried out exactly as the system instructs.

As more outbreaks and episodes of contaminated water supplies are linked to exposure to cow manure, there is growing interest in animal waste and its disposal, a problem exacerbated by intensive farming practices but a factor even where cattle graze naturally. As many as 40 to 60 percent of cattle herds have signs of infection. Officials in San Francisco are now very aware that grazing near one of that city's reservoirs may put the water at risk. Cattlemen are being asked to keep calves, which harbor the parasite more frequently, away from the reservoir. Regulations governing the production, storage, and disposal of animal wastes are needed, but may be a long time coming.

Cryptosporidium parvum

A parasitic protozoan.

Illness: Cryptosporidiosis

Signs and symptoms: Profuse, watery diarrhea, possibly with nausea, abdominal pain, vomiting, and low-grade fever

Onset time: 2 to 14 days after ingestion of the oocysts

Average duration of illness: In healthy individuals, usually not more than 2 weeks but occasionally as long as 6 weeks. In the immunocompromised the diarrhea may continue indefinitely.

Severity: Mild to moderate in the healthy; can be severe in the immunocompromised

Fatality rate: Depends on the health status of the infected individual. The fatality rate among those with AIDS may be as high as 55 percent.

Foods at particular risk of contamination: Water, apple cider, or foods contaminated after cooking. Raw milk, raw sausage and offal are possible sources, and fruits and vegetables are potential vehicles.

Nonfood sources: Swimming pools and lakes, person-to-person transmission, contact with infected animals

Treatment: Simply supportive measures to deal with symptoms. There is no FDA-approved therapy or even a standard of care. Antibiotics are usually ineffective, but one agent, paromomycin, has been shown in controlled studies to slightly reduce parasite numbers and decrease stool frequency, and it may lead to treatments that could speed repair of disrupted intestinal barrier function. Some studies in AIDS patients have shown spiramycin, used in Canada and Europe against the protazoan *Toxoplasma gondii,* to be effective against the infection in some individuals. Another study showed it to be ineffective, but there were questions about whether the medication was properly absorbed in oral form. In all studies some patients experienced adverse side effects.

GIARDIA LAMBLIA

Nancy Allen is an organic farmer and a Green Party spokesperson in Surry, Maine. A few years ago she and a group of environmental activists were meeting in the nearby town of Ellsworth in the Federal Building, which had rooms available for groups. A thirsty member of the group went to look for a usable tap and found one. Several people took a drink. Only later did they notice the tiny sign on the wall saying not to drink the water.

Not long afterward Nancy began having recurring bouts of diarrhea and felt generally awful, nauseated and without appetite. She was losing weight and the diarrhea would seem to get better then get worse again. Finally her doctor diagnosed her as having giardiasis, or infection with *Giardia lamblia,* a protozoan. In the meantime she had discovered that others in the group were suffering the same symptoms. She thought she knew where they'd picked up the bug.

The town seemed uninterested, perhaps as a defensive maneuver, but there were many cases of *Giardia* in the area. A few years later the town's water source would be changed. Allen received treatment for giardiasis, but even with medical attention it was a year before she was feeling herself again. Experiences can vary. Quick treatment can reduce the illness to a few weeks. Without it the illness runs its course, or it can wax and wane.

While anyone can pick up *Giardia,* the immunocompromised are particularly at risk for illness. In time, most people with healthy immune systems get over the infection even without treatment, although some may become asymptomatic carriers. In fact, the infection is so common that 25 percent of Americans with gastrointestinal disease test positive.

Giardia is a parasite, a teardrop-shaped protozoan that lives in the guts of warm-blooded animals and humans and can pass from infected feces into water or food. It can exist in a cyst form that protects it from adverse conditions, and it can survive for some time outside a host and in water. Because it is common in those who drink from streams or ponds while hiking or camping and because it is present in wild animals, it is sometimes called "beaver fever."

The water in Ellsworth is treated with chlorine, but the levels of chlorine normally used in drinking water won't always kill *Giardia,* which is tough and resistant, more so than bacteria or other parasites. A combination of ozone treatment, expensive filtration, and chlorination is the generally accepted approach for water treatment facilities, and under the new standards of the Clean Water Act more cities and town are adopting filtration, but many smaller systems still use only chlorination.

In the summer of 1998, Sydney, Australia, had to issue a boiled-water alert for nearly a week when both *Giardia* and *Cryptosporidium* were found in the water supply. Waste from infected animals was first thought to be the source—dead dogs were actually found in a canal supplying water—but another possibility was that pathogens in the environment from animal waste were carried by heavy rains after a prolonged dry spell and might well have flooded the system. Sewage leaks are another common source of contamination, as *Giardia* is routinely found in human sewage.

The question is, How did this pathogen come out of nowhere, so to speak, to lurk as a potential contaminant of public drinking water most would consider safe? Is water more contaminated today, or is the parasite simply attracting more attention? Probably both are happening. The intensive farming of food animals creates vast supplies of concentrated manure that may contain the protozoan.

Giardia was only identified as a human pathogen by the World Health Organization in 1981, but in areas where the source of clean drinking water is undependable, infection may be almost universal. Travelers are at risk of picking up the infection, and in any recurring case of diarrhea that does not respond to antibiotics, *Giardia* should be suspected, although it is perfectly possible to contract the illness at home. A number of cities have had widespread outbreaks.

Certainly public water departments that now supply millions may infect masses of people if they get contaminated. Thus widespread outbreaks will become more visible. The growing popularity of outdoor sports such as hiking, camping, and rock climbing means that more people may be tempted to drink from what appear to be pristine mountain streams but which may nevertheless be fouled by waste. And as more children who are not toilet trained or not proficient in bathroom and hand-washing skills attend day-care or nursery school, the parasite is likely to spread. So, just as with other food- or waterborne diseases, changes in culture and lifestyle are playing a role in the increased visibility and infection rate in developed countries.

When an outbreak occurs, sometimes the question is not what to do if you are infected, but what to do if you are not. Nancy Allen's daughter, Sara Goldberg, lives with her husband and two children in South Portland, Maine. Three days a week she works in a doctor's office, and on those days her youngest child, Ruby, attends the same day-care facility her older brother once attended. It is small, and Sara likes the owner and knows the other mothers and children well. One morning when she was dropping Ruby off, she noticed very few children at the facility. Then she overheard one of the mothers asking the owner if she was feeling any better. Inquiring, she found that the owner had been suffering with diarrhea, nausea, and loss of appetite for weeks. Her doctor attributed it to stress, but he had suggested she submit a stool sample. She told Sara she was going to have it done. She mentioned that several other children were out with diarrhea as well. Sara left Ruby, but she was worried. The following week she learned that the owner's stool samples had come back positive for *Giardia*. Two of the other children tested positive as well. The owner's physician told her to stop working, and she took a week off, but one of the positive children was not told to stay away. The child attended while infected but untreated. Alarmed, Sara decided to take Ruby out of school and keep her at home for a while; her sister was able to take over child-care duties. Later she would learn that the state epidemiologist's office does not advise closing day-care facilities during an outbreak because parents who have to work are tempted to take their possibly infected children to other day-care facilities where they could spread the infection. The office does recommend that children be screened for the parasite and those who test positive be treated.

Sara remembers that Ruby's day-care center later did shut completely for a week during which everything was disinfected. Parents of children who were infected were told not to bring them back until the doctor said they were free of the parasite. Fortunately the other parents were also able to keep their children at home rather than find another facility.

Ruby never became ill, and everyone else recovered nicely, but the situation brings up the perplexing choices that face a parent whose child is *not* ill. *Giardia* is a problem in child-care facilities that is unlikely to go away. Maine is experiencing a virtual epidemic of giardiasis in young children. It is not alone. A public health official in New Mexico says the situation is epidemic there as well; in fact, she says, infection with *Giardia* is the chief cause of "failure to thrive" in young children in her area. The situation is a new reality that parents must be prepared to face.

Giardia lamblia

A one-celled, teardrop-shaped, parasitic protozoan that moves using flagella and lives in the small intestines of warm-blooded mammals throughout the world.

Illness: Giardiasis

Signs and symptoms: Abdominal cramping; nausea; watery, yellowish, and foul-smelling diarrhea; bloating and gas; weight loss; may trigger malabsorption (such as lactose intolerance)

Onset time: 1 to 2 weeks after ingestion of cysts; not everyone will show symptoms. Infected individuals may become asymptomatic carriers.

Average duration of illness: 4 to 6 weeks, although symptoms may continue to wax and wane.

Severity: Mild to moderate

Fatality rate: Low

Foods at particular risk of contamination: Water, foods made from contaminated water or foods washed in or otherwise contaminated by water containing cysts. Suspected water should be boiled for several minutes—longer at high altitudes.

Nonfood sources: Person-to-person contact. Outbreaks are frequent in day-care settings.

Treatment: Metronidazole (Flagyl) for adults; furazolidone (Furoxone) for children. Treatment is controversial as it may be worse than the disease; not everyone is treated.

WORMS

No one likes to think about worms in connection to what they are eating, and indeed the possibility of confronting one is not especially high. Sushi or other raw or undercooked fish dishes are the most likely source of an assortment of potential wiggly and unpleasant villains belonging to the anisakid nematode family. For that reason Japan has more cases, but as the popularity of sushi grows here in the United States, the incidence may increase. Among the specific worms: *Anisakis simplex, Hysterothylacium, Contracaecum* spp., and *Pseudoterranova decipiens*. Familiarly, *Anisakis simplex* is called the herring worm, and *Pseudoterranova decipiens,* the cod worm. When one of these critters produces disease in humans it is usually referred to as anisakiasis. Fewer than 60 cases have been reported in the United States, but many more probably go unreported. One estimate is that there are about 10 cases a year.

The symptoms of harboring one of these worms are no more pleasant than the thought. People report a tickling sensation in the throat, and coughing may bring up a worm that can then be extracted with the fingers. Other times there may be nausea and pain that can feel like appendicitis. The pain can come from the worm burrowing into the wall of the digestive tract, sometimes penetrating the intestinal wall and wandering around in the body cavity. Eventually the body responds, forming a granuloma—a chronically inflamed mass of tissues—around the worm.

The length of time between ingesting a worm and experiencing symptoms varies from an hour to two weeks. It may be comforting to know that roundworms don't usually grow to full maturity in humans and are likely to be eliminated within three weeks of infection. But old worm infections can apparently still produce pain.

Finding and identifying the worm can be done quite simply if it is coughed up. Other cases may require use of a fiber optic device. A worm may be found because the symptoms mimic appendicitis, resulting in surgery. In one case, reliably reported in the *New England Journal of Medicine*, a young man experienced severe abdominal pain. Surgery was performed, and the physicians were about to suture up the abdomen when a pinkish red worm crawled out onto the drapery.

These parasites have been found in the flesh of a wide variety of common fish, such as Pacific salmon, cod, herring, flounder, monkfish, and haddock. Fish are frequently passed over a light table to inspect for these worms as they can easily be seen with the naked eye. While this is pretty effective with a white-fleshed fish, candling a fish such as salmon, which has colored flesh, may be more difficult. Thoroughly freezing fish for seven days before consuming it raw can kill the worm, but salmon is unsuited to this technique. Of course the worms are also killed by thorough cooking. (Although dead, they are still there, but consider it another source of protein. I'm sure all of us fish eaters have consumed these dead worms occasionally and never noticed—thank goodness.)

There are other worms, such as *Ascaris lumbricoides* (common roundworm) and *Trichuris trichiura,* that can be found in food or transmitted by infected food handlers. They come from using improperly treated sewage as fertilizer. The eggs of the worms can survive in soil, and humans can become infected when they eat raw vegetables. Individuals may not know they are infected unless worms are noticed in their feces.

Horribly, these worms may crawl up into the throat and attempt to get out of the body through the nose or mouth. The larvae may migrate into the lungs and cause a kind of pneumonia. Infestation with these worms can cause vague discomfort in the digestive tract, and in a small child the large worms may cause a blockage. They can be found around the world, but *Ascaris* is more common in North America, and *Trichuris,* in Europe. Sometimes infection with the worms is self-resolving when the worms go through their life cycle. In other cases treatment with a vermifuge (worm-expelling drug) is called for or in severe cases, surgery.

According to FDA documents, eggs of *Ascaris* spp. have been found in cabbage, but any uncooked vegetables and fruit growing in or around untreated sewage are vulnerable. It is assumed that there are many more cases than those reported because routine tests of sewage in the United States have revealed a significant number of eggs, implying a high infection rate.

An extremely rare worm infection can occur with *Eustrongylides,* a bright red roundworm. These worms are found in raw or under-cooked fish. They attach to the wall of the digestive tract and can cause severe pain. The worms have a life cycle that moves from wading birds, where the larvae mature, to fresh-water, brackish-water, and marine fish. They continue to be very active even after the death of the fish. A risk factor is eating whole minnows, but one case was reported from eating sashimi. These worms should be easy to spot in raw fish, but it's well to point out that in the sashimi case the raw fish was prepared at home. Experienced sushi and sashimi preparers are more likely to know what to look for.

Diphyllobothrium latum is a tapeworm or broad fish flatworm. Infection with it is rare, but it can follow consumption of infected, undercooked freshwater fish. The symptoms are gas, bloating, and diarrhea; they occur about 10 days after eating the fish.

The message of all these pests seems to be that eating under-cooked or raw fish should be undertaken with extreme caution, and that all vegetables should be thoroughly washed before eating.

Worms

Various parasitic worms found in fish, contaminated soil, or water pose health threats to humans through ingestion of common foods. They are generally rare, and the symptoms vary with the worm. Check the preceding text for details. See a physician if you suspect you are infected.

BOVINE SPONGIFORM ENCEPHALOPATHY

The story of mad cow disease, more properly known as bovine spongiform encephalopathy (BSE), is one of the most intriguing and compelling ever to emerge from the annals of medicine. It is a medical detective story; it involves politics, economics, agriculture, science, and human behavior; and finally it is a tragedy. Mad cow disease, as it will forever be called, despite the earnest efforts of the beef industry to have the public refer to it by its difficult but correct name, has become a stunning potential epidemic event that has awakened the public—at least in the United Kingdom and Europe—and the industry, albeit not completely, to the inherent dangers of specific intensive agricultural practices. It has undermined further the confidence people once had in their government, their farmers, their agricultural specialists, their scientists, and indeed their food. And while no mad cows have yet been reported in the United States by the Department of Agriculture, the disease has had a significant impact in America, though much of it remains behind the scenes. In trade and medical journals, on web sites devoted to the disease, and within the worldwide community of food safety and public health officials, there is the quiet acknowledgment that problems related to transmissible spongiform encephalopathies, as diseases of this type are called, have really just begun.

The story begins in England in 1984 when David Bee, a veterinarian from Midhurst, West Sussex, was called to treat a cow acting oddly. It had lost weight, held an odd posture, trembled, was antisocial, and did not respond to treatment. Other cows on the farm began showing similar symptoms as the first cow worsened, its head tremors becoming constant. It died in February 1985. Over the next month the farmer lost 9 cows to the strange malady. In desperation he allowed a tenth to be sacrificed and its brain was sent to Central Veterinary Laboratory in Weybridge, Surrey, where it was examined in September by Carol Richardson, the pathologist on duty. She found small holes or vacules that she labeled "spongiform encephalopathy" in her report. She has seen the same holes in the brains in sheep that had died of scrapie and in subsequent interviews she recalled how excited she was to see the signs of the illness in a cow. (Keep in mind that pathologists become "excited" over things that might appall the rest of us, the oddness of the discovery being the cause.) In April of 1985 in England a forty-three-year-old Kent veterinarian, Colin Whitaker, had been called to look at a sick cow. Jonquil, as the cow was called, was usually good-natured, but her mood had changed. "She was behaving oddly," Whitaker remembers. She was nervous and aggressive and seemed apprehensive. He found she had cystic ovaries, which he treated, but nothing else that he could determine. The next time he checked on her she was worse. "Unsteady on her feet and very unhappy," he says. He thought of a number of explanations, but none seemed to fit. Eventually the animal was destroyed and its carcass sold for pet food. He remained puzzled, but thought of it as a "one-off" case. Then he began seeing more cases like Jonquil's in the same herd. He thought of possibilities such as a brain tumor or an illness called staggers. When he was contacted about the third cow, he knew it was no coincidence, and he too sent the brain to the Weybridge Lab, where an analysis set off an investigation that is ongoing to this day. But it would be 1999 before the earlier cases spotted by Bee and analyzed by Richardson would be linked publicly to Whitaker's, which obviously implies that the outbreak had begun earlier than generally supposed. It seemed clear that unrecognized cases had probably occurred elsewhere in the country, possibly as early as 1984. Today the investigation has involved hundreds and perhaps thousands of researchers worldwide, has intrigued and horrified scientists, and has badly shaken the beef industry, farmers, and consumers. Some suggest that the defeat of Britain's Conservative government in 1997 can be laid, at least partially, on its poor handling of what would turn out to be a significant threat to the public health.

What researchers would begin to unravel when they first looked at the brains of these sick animals—and many more would turn up—was a disease in which the brain developed a spongy-looking pattern of holes. As it progressed, the cows, like Jonquil, would develop tremors, aggressiveness, clumsiness, and fearfulness, eventually collapse, and have to be destroyed. The researchers also discovered that what linked the sick animals—and they looked at many different factors—was the consumption of feed containing rendered animal protein.

Responding to the pressures on farmers to make animals grow faster and, in the case of dairy cattle, to produce more milk, feed producers add protein to their product. It can come from plant or animal sources, and whichever is cheaper will generally be used by feed manufacturers. The first thought among investigators was that the disease, as Richardson had suspected, looked like scrapie, which has been around for 200 years, and indeed, dead scrapie-infected sheep had been rendered and recycled into animal feed. But what was making the outbreak worse was that dead mad cows were being rendered and fed back to animals as well, which effectively not only recycled the disease but very likely strengthened its virulence.

It is not certain today whether it was the initial inclusion of scrapie-infected sheep that set off the epidemic, or whether the condition is a rare, sporadic disease in cattle that had simply never been identified. It is very certain that recycling the diseased cattle into feed for animals and pets spread the infection. As the epidemic spread among cows, the big question in the minds of the British public was, Could people get sick from eating the meat of these animals?

At first, government experts were reassuring and said it could not. There was a "species barrier" between animals and humans, as far as disease was concerned. And there is a similar kind of fatal dementia in humans known as Creutzfeldt-Jakob disease, or CJD, that makes the brain look something like the cows' brains, but it has been around quite a while and is rare and apparently sporadic. In fact, transmissible spongiform encephalopathies (TSEs) have been identified in a number of groups of animals, such as North American elk and mink, and in the most bizarre case, among Papua New Guinea Fore tribespeople with a ritual practice of eating the dead—including the brain. The disease, studied by Dr. D. Carleton Gajdusek, who subsequently won a Nobel Prize for his work on TSEs, is called kuru, and when the cannibalistic practices were stopped, the disease gradually faded away.

There was no link between CJD and consuming British beef, since the disease appeared around the world. But based on the possibility that consuming BSE-infected beef could affect humans, the government began to regulate what parts of the animals went into human foods. Researchers had already discovered that some parts—

the spinal column, the eyes, the brain—were more dangerous and infectious than others. And some of these parts, to the surprise of consumers, were going into sausage and hamburger. Rules were adopted to stop that practice, but years later researchers would discover the rules had been ineffective. Unsavory bits and pieces of the animals were finding their way into ground meats just as they had been for as long as meat had been commercially ground.

What was worrying to the public—and to researchers—was that zoo animals and cats had begun turning up with a similar illness. Presumably it was from the food they were getting. Jonquil, after all, had been slaughtered for pet food. Apparently the infectious agent was being spread around. More worrying still, several farmers came down with CJD. But those scientists who raised warnings about the potential for a human epidemic from consuming infected beef were branded as alarmists. Even as the government was trying to still public fears and restore confidence in British beef, researchers were carrying out different sorts of studies. A special team of scientists was keeping a close watch on cases of an illness that had begun appearing in the United Kingdom that was like classic CJD and yet was not. The patients were younger, for one thing. Their disease didn't progress as quickly. It began with psychological symptoms. Their brains looked, not like classic CJD patients' brains, but more like those from the mad cows.

One of these patients was Victoria Rimmer, who lived with her grandmother in North Wales. An active young woman, Vicky, who loved animals, owned an English springer spaniel and in the evenings and weekends worked at a nearby kennel. She was 15 in June 1993 when her symptoms began. One day she simply disappeared and when she reappeared couldn't remember where she had been or what she had done. She was constantly tired, had trouble with her eyesight, experienced a growing clumsiness, and was losing weight. By August she had to be hospitalized. A specialist diagnosed her condition as CJD. She was the youngest person in the United Kingdom ever to contract the disease. Although Vicky's grandmother didn't know it at the time, there were now nine similar cases in the country. When a CJD expert from the government surveillance unit in Edinburgh that had been set up to track the emerging cases came down to see Vicky, he tried to talk her grandmother into keeping quiet about her condition. "He told me to think of what I was doing to Britain's economy," she later told a reporter, Peter Silverton of the *Mail on Sunday*. "I knew then that they had something to hide," she said. "It made me determined to find out how Vicky got the disease and to try and get the government to admit people could get mad cow disease."

On March 20, 1996, the British government, which had repeatedly reassured its people that there was no danger from consuming British beef, did a turnaround. An ashen-faced health secretary, Stephen Dorrell, announced that consumption of meat contaminated with BSE was "the most likely explanation at present" for a group of similar illnesses in humans. The reaction was devastating to the British beef industry. The British government first proposed slaughtering and incinerating 800,000 animals. However, carrying out any such cattle massacre would prove an enormous, almost impossible challenge. There weren't enough incineration facilities to handle the volume. And the proposed slaughter increased almost daily. Millions of animals might have to go to restore the reputation of British beef. (By 1998 the actual number slaughtered would be less than 200,000.)

While the public position of the U.S. beef industry was that the BSE-CJD connection could not be proved, the rest of the world was deeply concerned. An immediate ban on the importation of cattle from the United Kingdom was put into place by the European Union (EU), not only to protect its people but also its beef industry. Beef consumption was dropping daily; even the British McDonald's was advertising veggie burgers. EU officials also banned the importation of embryos, semen, and beef by-products including gelatin and tallow. Beef by-products, which had the potential to carry the infectious agent—thought to be a strange protein particle called a prion—went into candy, foods, cosmetics, drugs, and even medical appliances. They seemed to be everywhere and in everything. Adding to the problem, studies had demonstrated that the infectious agent was almost impossible to destroy. Ordinary methods of disinfecting and sterilization didn't affect it. Conceivably it could survive even the intense processing gelatin went through. Around the world breeding cattle from Britain were destroyed. In England itself officials began the horrible task of destroying animals, although most of them appeared perfectly healthy.

The World Health Organization recommended that ruminant-to-ruminant feeding be stopped, and the FDA began considering what changes it would make in U.S. rendering practices. The USDA and the National Cattlemen's Beef Association rushed to assure U.S. consumers that there were no dangers here. No beef had been imported from the United Kingdom since 1985, consumers were informed. But had beef gone to Italy and ended up in sausages that had been imported into the United States? Had cattle been shipped to South Africa and their remains used to make bone meal that had found its way to the United States? The fact was, no one really knew. World trade was too complex.

It would be almost a year before additional research provided a more conclusive link between BSE and England's new variant strain of CJD—or nvCJD, as it was now called. In October 1996 John Collinge and his team published reports of experiments that revealed the nvCJD strain to be genetically different from other types of CJD and more like those of BSE as transmitted to mice, domestic cats, and macaque monkeys. This finding was "consistent with BSE being the source of this new disease," the article said. Other studies made the link as well. But by then the doubters were quieter. Mad cow disease had changed the world and how we look at food and animal production. It had revealed the numerous foods, cosmetics, drugs, medical appliances, and other common objects that contain beef or beef by-products, many of which were now suspect as possible sources of the infectious agent. One looming question remained. Did Americans have anything to fear? When Howard Lyman, a participant on an Oprah Winfrey show, noted, among other things, that the same conditions—cows being fed cows—existed in the United States, both he and Winfrey were sued by cattlemen in Texas. Eventually the defendants won, but the cattlemen appealed the case. Nonetheless, there is certainly no doubt that similar feeding practices were being followed in the United States.

There is also some evidence that this country might have its own strain of TSE in bovines. The story begins with an outbreak of transmissible mink encephalopathy (TME) in 1963 on a mink ranch in Canada. Researchers had noticed that TME looked a lot like sheep scrapie, but when they tried to transfer scrapie to mink using injections into the brain, they had not been very successful. The mink rancher said that sheep, in fact, had not been used as feed. The mink instead had eaten dead and "downer" cattle. In 1985 another outbreak occurred in which 60 percent of 7,300 animals on one Stetsonville, Wisconsin, ranch came down with the disease and died. Again the mink had been fed a diet exclusively of downer cows. At the University of Wisconsin a researcher named Dr. Richard F. Marsh thought of the earlier Canadian outbreak.

Sheldon Rampton and John Stauber have written a book called *Mad Cow U.S.A.* They report that Marsh remembers asking the farmer if he had fed the mink any "rabies negative" animals. These would have been cows that showed neurological symptoms but tested negative for rabies. "He knew the number right off," Marsh told them. "He told us that he had fed 17 rabies-negative cattle. He showed us his record-keeping system, and every one was precisely entered," Marsh said.

Other researchers had considered the possibility that downer cows might be a source for TME, but in 1985 Marsh attended a meeting of the United States Livestock Association and warned the group that he had evidence that mink could contract TME from eating downer dairy cattle. He didn't know it at the time, but BSE had already been spotted in England. "I tried to put them on the alert to look for such a disease in dairy cows," Marsh told reporter Joel McNair of *Agri-View.* The term "downer" covers a great many conditions. It simply means that a cow cannot get up for some reason. Often these animals go for pet food—although occasionally they have been known to make their way into hamburger. Marsh began a series of experiments. He took material from the brains of the TSM-inspected mink and injected it into the brains of healthy mink, mice, ferrets, monkeys, hamsters, and two Holstein bull calves. The mink became ill first, then the monkeys. Ten of the hamsters died. The calves died in months 18 and 19. The ferrets resisted the longest, except for the mice, which weren't affected.

Surprisingly, the disease in the calves did not look like that of Britain's mad cows. Instead, the calves simply collapsed, exactly as downer cows do. They also had only a mild pattern of spongy holes in the brain. Marsh then took material from the calves brains and injected it into healthy mink. The mink developed TME within four months.

Marsh surmised that if the mink on the Stetsonville ranch had contracted the illness by eating infected cattle, there may be an unrecognized TSE in cattle—one that looks different from both scrapie (in sheep) and the British BSE. Marsh concluded that if it existed, it was probably rare. But the origins of BSE in Great Britain had likely been equally as rare. The problem was that it didn't stay rare once the diseased animals began being recycled in the animal food chain.

The USDA has regularly tested cattle brains for mad cow disease and to date has reported discovering no incidences. While they began by looking for the British brain patterns, they now look for other possible signs as well. They have also begun to randomly check the brains of downer cows and to check the brains of those that are rabies-negative. All of this checking is spotty, however. They do not have the resources to check as thoroughly as they might like. Another problem is that dairy cows are slaughtered earlier in the United States than in the United Kingdom. It may well be that spent dairy cows are going to market long before they might be expected to show signs of the illness, and that even if they were older, the signs of the disease might be different—and thus go unrecognized.

Another issue involves whether the reported rates of Creutzfeldt-Jakob disease are accurate. Is it as rare as the CDC says—simply one in a million, or about 250 cases a year in the United States? Probably not. "The good news is that people may not be contracting Alzheimer's [disease] as often as we think," the audience of ABC's "World News Tonight" heard Peter Jennings say on May 12, 1997. "The bad news is that they may be getting something worse instead." An ABC reporter said that several autopsy studies suggest that CJD has been underdiagnosed. "The studies show that when pathologists actually did autopsies and examined brain tissue from patients with Alzheimer's and other brain disorders, they uncovered hidden cases of CJD. These preliminary findings suggest a public health problem is being overlooked. If larger autopsy studies at more hospitals confirmed that even 1 percent of Alzheimer's patients had CJD, that would mean 40,000 cases, and each undetected case is significant because, unlike Alzheimer's, CJD is infectious."

It is not surprising that CJD is underdiagnosed. The disease is known to be highly infective in certain very specific ways. Instruments used in brain probes have transmitted the disease to other patients even after sterilization. Transplants of certain organs from patients who died of CJD have transmitted the disease. Some of the young people who received human growth hormone in the 1970s began coming down with the disease. The hormone was made from the pituitary glands of many individuals, some of whom had died of CJD. (Now a synthetic hormone is used.)

Thus both neurosurgeons and pathologists are reluctant to investigate too deeply patients with suspected CJD. In short, definitive diagnoses are sometimes not made, and autopsies are often not being performed when CJD is suspected—this according to both neurosurgeons and pathologists themselves.

The ABC report did not mention mad cows and the situation with British beef, and the danger that U.S. livestock and thus the beef supply were contaminated was played down—but the danger does exist. Several things are worrisome about the safety of the U.S. meat supply with regard to TSEs. One is that the ban against ruminant-to-ruminant feeding, enacted by the FDA after months of delay, does not go far enough. The FDA's regulation allows potentially TSE-positive materials to be used in pet food, and pig, chicken, and fish feed. "Thus, TSE-infected deer could legally be sent to the renderer and converted into pet and pig rations," wrote the food-safety researcher Michael Hanson in "The Reasons Why FDA's Feed Rule Won't Protect Us from BSE," an article that appeared in *Genetic Engineering News*, an industry publication. Another major question is whether renderers are able to keep feed containing potentially infectious material separated from feed destined for ruminants. It is difficult to know. The FDA says it has sufficient funds for enforcement. The FDA rule also exempts blood and blood products even though they are now seen in Great Britain as possible agents of infectivity. Finally, there are reports that the vacuum devices that clean every bit of meat off of the spinal column at slaughter facilities are picking up bits of spinal cord. This pastelike meat material is used in some processed meat products.

Dr. Gajdusek outlined for Richard Rhodes, author of *Deadly Feasts*, all the possible routes of infection in a world that uses these animals in hundreds of different ways. "It means your pigskin wallet. It means catgut surgical suture, because that's made of pig tissue. All the chickens fed on meat-and-bone meal: they're probably infected. You put the stuff in a chicken and it goes right through. A vegetarian could get it from chicken-shit that they put on the vegetables. It could be in the tallow, in butter—how the hell am I supposed to measure infectivity in the butter? . . . These people who've come down with CJD have given blood. It's undoubtedly in the blood supply. . . . And by the way, it could be in the milk."

Conclude Rampton and Stauber: "The number of hypothetical risks from these novel disease agents seems endless. . . . The experts tend to argue that each of these hypothetical avenues, taken individually, poses little danger. . . . Government and industry, officials worry that public discussion of hypothetical risks could trigger unnecessary panic. The truth is that the risks come from so many directions and are so unpredictable that consumers can't and shouldn't be expected to cope with those risks by selectively boycotting products suspected of harboring an unseen infection. There are too many bullets to dodge, and the shots may be blanks anyway. What we need is good data, and in the meantime we need serious implementation of measures to prevent the disease from spreading—*not* just surveillance that will only alert us to tragedy after it has already arrived."

It is now easy to see where Great Britain went wrong. Pressures from the beef industry meant that time was wasted in ensuring the safety of the food supply, thus endangering the health of an entire generation. It is still uncertain how many people will eventually develop nvCJD, but the transmission of BSE to humans clearly represents a betrayal of the public trust. At this writing 35 cases of this fatal illness have been confirmed, but no one thinks that is the end of it. One of the problems in the United Kingdom was seen, in hindsight, to have been the inherent conflict within the British Ministry of Agriculture, Fisheries, and Food (MAFF) to both promote agricultural products and regulate food safety. That same conflict exists in the United States today. The British are now creating a single food-safety agency. The United States should do the same.

But the food industry is expected to put up a fierce battle against any attempt to create such an agency, and the legislative bills introduced so far have gone nowhere.

Say Rampton and Stauber, "If we let industry set the rules, however, there will literally be no limit to what we'll swallow, and the nightmare of mad cow disease—or something just as bad, or worse—not only *can* happen here, but almost certainly *will*."

3

Avoiding Foodborne Disease

EATING OUT ON THE EDGE

When you eat away from home, the safety of your food is in someone else's hands. Never forget that. And those hands, in all probabil-
ity, belong to someone making minimum wage, who doesn't have
sick leave either. You cannot be sure they are clean hands, or that the
person they are connected to has had any training in food safety, or
even that the restaurant owner has a clear understanding of how
foodborne microbes get into food. In short, eating out, from a food-
safety perspective, involves risk. At worst, it can be a nightmare; at
best, it is an adventure.

Having researched and written about foodborne disease for five
years, I've moved from being a journalist to something I hadn't anticipated. At a conference a few years ago a friend told me that a
woman sidled up to him, pointed to me, and said, "Eat what she
eats." That's a big responsibility. I do eat carefully, applying what I
know. But I also take chances on occasion, just as we all do and just
as healthy people should. To go through life terrorized by the possibility of encountering foodborne microbes would be to make life
hardly worth living. When I do take risks, I make a series of fact-
based evaluations mixed with assorted subjective, sensory-based, and
intuitive judgments that are then combined with my cultural background, personal experience, and finally the mood I'm in. It's not an
entirely rational procedure, and it may not always work. Eating

safely is a complex business, and few of us act completely rationally—certainly not me. However, I cannot remember having a bout of gastrointestinal illness in a decade, while all around me I hear sad tales of unpleasant experiences. A healthy-looking young man told me he had experienced three serious bouts in recent years, one of which put him in the hospital. Quite unusually, the cause was identified in all three cases: *Salmonella, Shigella,* and *Campylobacter.* On a whim I asked him if he took antacids. "He gobbles them down," his wife said. I told him that from the perspective of foodborne disease he should therefore consider himself in the immune-impaired category, as the reduction of protective stomach acid by antacids can make a person more vulnerable.

Risk can be managed by how you select food when you are eating out. How much risk one wants to take is a personal decision. After all, some people like risk; rock climbing, skiing, and hang gliding are popular sports. Some of us also like food—a great deal—and there are times when a particular risk may seem worth it. I eat in restaurants, but I am careful about what I eat.

How much risk you want to take should depend on the state of your health, which only you really know. Factors to consider when evaluating your potential susceptibility to foodborne disease go beyond the obvious—and beyond taking antacids. They include being at the extremes of age (parents are obviously responsible for making decisions for their children, and guidance should certainly be given to some much older individuals so that they are not put at risk) and the status of one's immune system. Having just recovered from an illness, even a bad cold, or being treated with an antibiotic can increase an individual's risk of getting sick. Undergoing a cancer therapy, having AIDS, being a transplant recipient, having liver damage—all can make you very vulnerable.

Choosing a restaurant carefully is the first step in staying well. Common sense applies, and it is important to pay attention. If you know nothing else about a restaurant, dirty windows, weeds growing in cracks in the sidewalk in front, garbage strewn around the back entrance, and a messy or grimy look to the interior will tell you that cleanliness is not a high priority. One public health official uses the cleanliness of the bathroom as her clue to the restaurant's standards. An eating establishment that isn't careful to keep clean what its patrons can see won't be careful about what patrons can't see—you can be sure of that. On the other hand, a clean-looking fast-food restaurant can depend almost entirely upon a low-paid teenage workforce with a high employee turnover rate and thus have its food-safety vulnerabilities as well.

The quality of a restaurant can make a difference. The more expensive and the better the reputation a restaurant has, the more likely the chef will have had good training in food safety at a culinary institute. On the other hand, it is no guarantee. The most expensive restaurant may unknowingly purchase food already contaminated. The people who were infected with *Cyclospora* from raspberries in 1996 and 1997 generally ate then in expensive venues.

If you are looking for absolute guarantees in restaurant foods, there are none. In general, the old rule "Hot foods hot and cold foods cold" still applies. A dish meant to be hot, such as a stew, casserole, or lasagna, should be hot all the way through—steamy hot. Reheating in a microwave, as some restaurants do, can leave cold spots. If you discover these cold spots, send back whatever it is. Be bold.

In the past 20 years as diets have changed, raw fresh fruits and vegetables have become very popular. An epidemiologist tells of an outbreak at a university that was eventually linked to the salad bar. A great many of those sick were freshman women who ate virtually nothing but raw fruits and vegetables. "Ironically," he says, "the guys wolfing down the hamburgers, which were thoroughly cooked, were fine."

Just the thought of salad bars can bring a groan from an epidemiologist. If you're looking for a way to combine risk factors, they're all there in beautiful array, and numerous outbreaks have been traced to these popular buffets. The reason? The preparation of salad-bar items is extensive, and hands are all over everything as the peeling and chopping takes place. Cross-contamination can occur if vegetables are cut on a surface previously used to prepare raw meats. Foods may not be maintained at a proper temperature in a salad bar or breakfast bar. They are also vulnerable to contamination from customers. In outbreaks where the original source of contamination has been in only one of the foods in a buffet, it has sometimes been transferred to other food items as utensils have been switched by diners. If a salad bar or buffet is your only choice, go for foods that have had a heavy dose of vinegar (a microbe inhibitor), such as bean salads, or choose hot foods that are obviously hot. Absolutely avoid any that might be tempting for hands, such as bowls of loose raisins.

Avoiding buffet foods can be a greater challenge than one might imagine. Ask to be served cantaloupe and you may see the waiter go to the breakfast buffet to get it for you instead of cutting it fresh. Vigilance and determination are required.

The question of served salad, not from a salad bar but on a plate, is a more difficult one. Some epidemiologists think twice about uncooked salad greens, and a few avoid salads altogether. If the other signs are good, you may want to take a chance. If the chance is worth it—if you're desperate for fresh greens—go ahead knowingly, but you might consider avoiding alfalfa sprouts, which have caused several outbreaks recently. Wait for word that the sprout industry has found a way to decontaminate the seeds. They are working on this. If you are wondering what's available for that quick, nutritious lunch where previously a salad had been the answer, hot soups are a safer choice.

Sandwiches open the door to problems. Eating ready-made sandwiches out of cooler shelves and even machines is taking a chance. Blind faith in the unknown individuals who prepared these sandwiches is unwarranted. How were they transported? When were they made? Were they always kept refrigerated? There are too many unanswered questions for a careful eater. Anyone who thinks food inspectors are standing over the preparers should think again. Confidence of this sort is not just misplaced but verges on irrationality.

Hands that prepare sandwiches should be wearing gloves. In a café, make certain that people working the cash register are not preparing foods. If they are, go someplace else. Don't buy anything from a sidewalk vendor except roasted peanuts—in the shell.

All of us take risks on occasion. Seared tuna is especially tempting. But the less thoroughly animal products are cooked, the more danger there is in consuming them. In the case of raw or undercooked fish the danger is parasites—worms to be more precise. Fish needs to be not only absolutely fresh to be served as sushi but carefully inspected on a light table for these visible pathogens. Fortunately there are not many cases of parasitic infection in the United States from raw fish, but those who have had one don't want a repeat. Eat sushi if you will, but only in the best Japanese restaurant, one with a large Japanese clientele, since custom and experience are the best guides to safe foods. In Japan, where sushi preparers are certified, it's safer. Here there are no such assurances. Caution is the operative word.

Avoid ordering dishes that contain undercooked eggs. Ask how a dish is prepared if there is a question. Order your eggs hard cooked and ask that egg dishes be prepared from freshly broken eggs rather than "pooled" eggs, which is the cracking of many eggs together, a practice that allows one contaminated egg to taint the entire mixture.

Under no circumstances should anyone eat a less than thoroughly cooked hamburger. The nature of hamburger (see page 11) increases the risk of contamination being spread throughout the product, and the consequences of confronting *E. coli* O157:H7, even for healthy individuals, can be not just unpleasant but grim. Anyone eating a rare hamburger, no matter where, is being foolhardy.

Rare steak or pink lamb is something else entirely. The contamination associated with beef is on the outside; muscle meat is sterile until it is contaminated with fecal material, usually during the slaughtering or butchering process. Therefore, a steak or roast that hasn't been pierced or poked (which can spread the bacterial contamination to the interior), can be eaten rare because bacterial contamination on the surface will be killed. Again, this is something you have to ask about when you order a steak.

It is no longer a good idea to eat raw or undercooked shellfish anywhere. In the summer of 1998 a huge outbreak of foodborne disease was associated with shellfish from the Gulf of Mexico; the previous year the Northwest was implicated in a large outbreak. Well-cooked shellfish are still fine from a microbial perspective. (Of course, large fish from Caribbean or tropical waters can harbor toxins, but that is another matter.) Individuals with liver disease need to be extremely cautious about undercooked shellfish as they are more vulnerable to a common shellfish-borne pathogen.

If this seems to be a recipe for never eating out, think again. Even low-cost foods can be safe. A good pizza is about as sure a bet as you can get at the low end of the cost scale. The fast-food chains are extremely conscious of the danger of undercooked hamburger, and it is doubtful that you will ever see one at a major franchise. (Food quality and the long-term health consequences from eating fast food are not issues addressed in this book.) In a corner café or family restaurant, go for the meatloaf special with mashed potatoes, vegetable, and apple pie, all piping hot. Chinese and Indian restaurants where everything is hot and steamy are good bets, but to be really safe, avoid the fried rice. Thai restaurants, where some of the foods can be raw and freshly prepared, are a little riskier, but again, plenty of well-cooked choices are on these menus as well. On the pricier end of restaurant dining, have a hot soup, grilled or sautéed meat or fish, and vegetable and end up with a crème caramel or the brown Betty. Ice cream is almost always a safe choice.

Vegetarians have more of a problem. Pasta dishes are usually the answer. Vegans are hard-pressed to eat out anyway, but they already know this and are accustomed to coping. Don't be afraid to order off menu. Asking for rice and steamed vegetables is a safe solution for the vegan diner.

All of these rules apply equally to eating at friends' houses. Avoid the bowls of peanuts or other snack foods where everyone's hands have been. Don't eat caterer-prepared sushi. You have no idea if the caterer is expert or not, and no one is ever offended by people who refuse passed appetizers.

After that, things will be trickier. Friends are not the anonymous owners of restaurants, and friendship may be more important than avoiding the possibility of illness, but that's for you to judge. But if it's a helping-in-the-kitchen situation, you can always say, "I'll wash the lettuce," if you're not certain it would be done properly otherwise. It's perfectly acceptable to say that you want your hamburger well done, or even that you don't eat hamburger but are content with tomato on a bun. If you have other problems with something being served, especially at a sit-down dinner, it's best, for the sake of politeness, to be subtle about avoiding certain dishes unless you have a medical condition you don't mind mentioning. In that case you have permission to eat whatever you feel is appropriate, shunning openly what you feel is not. The risks become simply too great.

It should go without saying that dinnertime at other people's houses is not the place to bring up the question of unsafe foods, unless you see a two-year-old about to take a bite of a rare hamburger. Then it would be almost criminal not to intervene.

To all these rules there are exceptions. Well armed with facts, you're the boss.

TRAVELING WITH YOUR STOMACH

To travel, if it is not simply a part of business, is to set out in search of the unusual, the unexpected, and the unfamiliar, to intentionally expose yourself to change and challenge and difference. Yet there is often the paradoxical urge to try to avoid precisely those elements, for change and the unfamiliar always translate into increased risk.

Today it is possible to travel in a comfort bubble. The standard Americanized hotel suite has multiplied around the globe as if it were an aggressive organism. From the confines of a protected space with air-conditioning and hot and cold running water, the modern tourist can have it both ways, safely viewing other landscapes and cultures from, or retreating into, a protective shell.

Food is the last frontier. Unless you subsist on suitcases full of prepackaged, dehydrated meals, you must eat and drink several times a day, and that food and drink, precisely because it is different, will provide challenges to the body. Studies by experts in travel medicine have found that between 20 and 50 percent of all travelers experience what is called TD, or travelers diarrhea. Other studies show that having a bout of disease affects the perceived "quality of life," another way of saying that whether you enjoy yourself and have good memories of the trip may depend on your staying well.

Travelers diarrhea, a catch-all term, refers to foodborne disease from all the familiar sources as well as a few that aren't normally confronted on home turf. Avoiding the phenomenon doesn't require a custom-designed program for particular foodborne pathogens, except in rare cases (see Ciguatera and Other Fish Toxins in chapter 2). Just a few general food-safety techniques can help prevent an unpleasant experience.

TD can be quirky. In a group of six acquaintances who had rented a villa in Italy for an extended stay, only one became ill, and yet he couldn't think what he had eaten that the others had not eaten. In fact, what can make one individual ill might bypass another. Anyone who knows he or she is more vulnerable for whatever reason should take precautions. And yet, slipups are easy. A seasoned traveler friend thought she was being careful on a trip to Central America but came down with a serious parasitic infection on her return. The only risk she could remember taking was brushing her teeth with tap water.

In most cases what causes an illness will remain a mystery. Occasionally the source can be discovered. Travelers to Latin America were made ill by crabs contaminated with *Vibrio cholerae* that they had brought back during the height of the epidemic there. It should be a given that perishable food be left behind.

Foodborne disease can strike even the most safety conscious. One expert in foodborne disease, an acknowledged authority on *Campylobacter, Helicobacter pylori,* and *Salmonella typhi,* was visiting India a few years ago on return from doing *Campylobacter* studies in Pakistan. He spent the day walking around in the sun and found himself profoundly thirsty. Knowing what he knew about foodborne disease risks, he looked around for something safe to drink and found nothing. Then he spotted a watermelon. It had not been cut and thus the presumably uncontaminated interior promised safety. And it would quench his thirst. He bought a freshly cut slice and ate it hungrily.

His trip took him to England, where he visited with another *Campylobacter* expert, and then he set out for home. He had already begun to feel ill. At home he struggled on for a day, then had to give in to the illness that had overtaken him. He was feverish and incredibly weak. When his wife insisted he go to the hospital—and he agreed by this time—he had to be wheeled in. He knew what he had. All the signs of typhoid fever were present. To his advantage he knew exactly how to treat it and could help the doctors, who were unfamiliar with an illness that is now relatively rare in the United States. He recovered.

Still, he was puzzled about where he had picked up the bug until a colleague more familiar with India told him that eating the watermelon was exactly the wrong thing to do. Watermelons are sold by weight, and water, which will add weight, can be injected into a

melon with no obvious signs on the outside. That may well have
been the source of his illness.

This is a discouraging story. If a foodborne disease expert can
pick up a foodborne illness unsuspectingly, what hope is there for
the average traveler? Still, watermelon is a unique fruit because of its
high water content. The old advice to "peel it, boil it, cook it, or
forget it" still holds.

The degree to which this is applied will depend on the country
and the perception of risk. Most people do not follow these rules in
the United States, even though much of the fresh produce is imported from around the globe. Perhaps they should, but risk is perceived as not that great, and it probably actually isn't that great
when one considers the mathematical chance of getting sick at any
particular meal, which is likely to be low.

Similar low risks would apply in Europe, Canada, New Zealand,
Japan, Australia, and other developed countries. The danger rises
when sanitation levels seem inadequate. Avoiding salad is, for instance, the only reasonable thing to do in some countries; it is less of
a risk in others. But it remains a risk, however small, even here in
the United States.

Eating the food of other countries is a big part of travel and one
of the chief pleasures for many. It is another way of getting to know
a country, a way to actually "taste" a culture. Whether you want to
take a risk will depend upon the state of your general health and the
importance of remaining well. Are you on a business trip where an
illness could mean an economic disaster or just traveling for pleasure? These are decisions that only you can make. Some taste sensa-
tions may be worth the risk, but any such encounters should be
undertaken consciously, knowing and understanding the risks with
a willingness to suffer the consequences.

Well-cooked foods that arrive at the table hot are unlikely to
cause problems. All raw foods, on the other hand, are suspect in areas where sanitation and hygiene are suspect. If you eat fruit, wash it
first, then peel it yourself. Avoid raw milk or cheeses made from it.
Raw or undercooked shellfish and meat can carry pathogens; to reduce your risks, avoid them and choose cooked dishes. Cooked
foods that have sat at room temperature should be thoroughly reheated. Look for steam as a sign of thorough heating. Eating from

street vendors can be risky anywhere but is downright foolhardy in areas where sanitation is not up to par. If you must, look for items cooked thoroughly before your eyes.

Interestingly, food scientists have increasingly noted that it is probably no accident that people in hot climates, where the threat of foodborne disease is greater, tend to eat spicy foods. Studies reveal that hot peppers contain a substance that kills bacteria. Combine hot peppers with vinegar and you have added a safety margin, but not a guarantee.

Any change in water, which will mean a change in the microbial communities that exist in all water, can cause a mild intestinal upset. If you want a general rule for travel, it is wise to drink one brand of bottled water whenever you travel, even in the United States. And don't allow restaurants to serve it with ice, which will have been made from tap water.

Chlorination will kill most microbes, but *Giardia, Cryptosporidium,* and *Entamoeba histolytica,* which causes amebic dysentery, can survive. If water and general sanitation are a concern, drink only tea or coffee made with boiled water; canned and bottled soft drinks including carbonated water and beverages (open these yourself or see that they are opened in front of you); or wine and beer. Potentially contaminated water should not be mixed in beverages, used to make ice, or even used to brush teeth. Do not allow ice to be served with canned or bottled drinks, and if a container has held ice, it should be thoroughly washed with soap and water before being used for drinking. In fact, drinking directly from a can or bottle is safer than using a questionable glass or mug. Since water on the outside of a bottle or can may be contaminated, dry or wipe containers clean before drinking from them.

Boiling water for one full minute (three minutes if you are at an altitude higher than 6,500 feet), then allowing it to cool naturally to room temperature (do not add ice), is the best guarantee of safe water. Aerating it by pouring back and forth or adding a pinch of salt to a quart will help the taste. If you can't boil water, it can be treated with chemicals. Tincture of iodine from the medicine cabinet or first-aid kit can be added at five drops to a quart (doubled if the water is cloudy). If the water is very cold or very cloudy, let it stand for several hours if possible. Commercially prepared tablets are available from sporting goods and camping stores, camping catalogs, and pharmacies. Use them according to directions.

Traveling with an infant will mean special problems most easily avoided if the child is breast-fed. A weaned infant can be given powdered formula or dry infant cereal mixed with boiled water; it should be eaten at once.

Certain kinds of travel bring certain kinds of risks. A number of outbreaks have been linked to food served on airplanes. It is subject to the factors that make large outbreaks possible: mass production and the chance that the food will suffer "temperature abuse" and then be inadequately reheated or served without further heating. Because travelers go in all directions after getting off a plane and may not consider what they ate on the plane as a source of subsequent illness, there are probably many more actual outbreaks then are ever reported and investigated. Many savvy travelers do not eat at all on plane trips but merely drink bottled water. That's not a bad idea. And as more airlines cut back on what they serve, the question of whether to eat or not may be irrelevant. But to be certain of what you are eating on a short trip, bring your own food prepared at home.

Cruises are another matter altogether. Eating is considered an important part of the experience, but epidemiologists who have investigated the many outbreaks of foodborne disease on these vessels call them "floating salad bars," for the reasons that epithet implies. There is a correlation between the general sanitation of a vessel and the chances of an outbreak. The CDC monitors vessel sanitation, and before booking a cruise it is smart to check out their Green Sheet, which lists inspection scores and boats that have failed to pass. It is available either by mail, fax, or on the Web. Pick a clean ship. Then if you want a further advantage, avoid the seafood salad. No single item pops up as a source of foodborne disease on these vessels more frequently, although other foods, such as potato salad and even sprouts, have caused outbreaks. Water can be another problem on cruise ships. The water supply can become contaminated, spreading illness throughout the boat. To be safe, drink only bottled water and brush your teeth with it.

For short trips by car, taking your own food is a tradition that should be revived. Healthy and safe foods that are better and cheaper than what you are likely to find on the road can be prepared at home. It can be as simple as hard-boiled eggs and tomatoes, or sandwiches and bottled drinks, or it can be more elaborate. When I was a child and my family traveled in Europe, lunch was the best part of the day. We would stop for cheese, good bread, fruit, and sliced luncheon meats and have a feast. A simple and otherwise boring journey can be turned into an event with a little planning. My grandmother always prepared fried chicken, bread-and-butter sandwiches, and deviled eggs for a day's journey, and the gesture was highly appreciated. A look at the map can reveal where there are scenic overlooks, and a meal stop can be planned to take advantage of one, thus combining food you know is safe with something more interesting than the generic interstate fast-food rest stops. But be certain to keep perishable foods cool in some sort of insulated container and wash all fruit before packing it.

Hands are a source of foodborne pathogens, and when traveling it may not always be convenient to wash before eating. But it may be more important than ever. It's a good idea to carry a hand disinfectant along. New products are appearing on the market daily. Prepackaged wipes now have disinfecting ingredients. A good supply of moistened paper towels in a Ziploc bag is better than nothing. When traveling with children, keep a supply in the car for snack times (and other emergencies).

When traveling in areas where diarrhea is a real possibility, take along packets of oral rehydration solution. There are prophylactic products on the market, but none has been shown to be very effective. Except for hepatitis A and cholera, there are no vaccines against the foodborne diseases you might confront, and the cholera vaccine is not particularly effective. Avoidance is the best medicine.

BUYING, STORING, AND PREPARING FOODS

People who pay close attention to press warnings about contaminated food often come away with the terrible feeling that there is nothing safe left to eat. It is important to correct that impression. Avoiding foodborne disease forces us to pay more attention to what we eat; it doesn't mean we can't enjoy food. In fact, in the long run, giving our food the attention that it deserves, knowing where it comes from, who has prepared it, and how it is prepared, and insisting on safer food will make eating more pleasurable than ever. Even in the short run, being careful doesn't mean abandoning pleasure in foods—as any kosher, halaal, or macrobiotic cook could tell you.

In the past few years there have been enough outbreaks and recalls to convince most people that foodborne disease is a very real problem. Familiar foods have changed. What were safe choices a generation or even a decade ago are no longer safe choices today. The old approaches to food weren't necessarily wrong, they simply no longer apply. How we are producing (growing and raising), processing, and distributing foods have all changed in the last generation. As consumers our expectations for variety, availability, convenience, and price have changed. In the process we have opened doors to emerging foodborne pathogens.

The new awareness of foodborne disease is not limited to consumers. The USDA has joined forces with the Departments of Health and Human Services and Education, the Food Marketing Institute, and a host of food associations such as the American Meat Institute and the American Egg Board to bring food-safety information to the public. The campaign is called Fight Bac, and it can be accessed on the World Wide Web. This sort of public-private partnership is seen as an effective way to do business in an age of tight budgets. It is also a good way to make certain that the message is shaped to fit the interests of those who are paying for it. The information is generally accurate, but it is subtly slanted to put consumer products in the best light possible, downplaying the dangers in some cases, and it should be read with that in mind. The USDA and the FDA also have their own web sites where there is excellent information, and they also have hot lines for specific consumer problems, but they no longer distribute free literature on a regular basis.

The family grocery buyer is the front line of safe food at home. The old skills of careful shopping need to be revived. You are about to spend your money on food for your family or yourself. You must be professional in your approach, knowing a great deal about the foods you are about to purchase, making no assumptions about safety or freshness. Be a dragon in the food market: competent and knowledgeable, endlessly curious, consistently demanding, and eternally vigilant.

PRODUCE

Food should certainly not be spoiled or dangerous, but neither should it be substandard in any other way. Produce should not just look fresh, because it has been gassed, waxed, irradiated, stored, or packaged under modified atmospheric conditions (where the oxygen that can promote spoilage has been removed and replaced with other gases), it should actually be fresh. Leafy vegetables should look "sprightly," with a certain vibrancy in their leaves. There is an "alive" look to produce that you can train your eye to recognize (or that your eyes already know, if you can begin again to have confidence in them). It has to do with color, brightness, and a certain tension. "Trust your senses," advises the Produce Marketing Association, and they are right. To quote Dr. Benjamin Spock, "You know more than you think you do."

Why is freshness so important? It means enhanced vitamin content for one thing; for another, signs of spoilage (caused by bacteria) can also indicate that other, pathogenic organisms may have contaminated the product and had an opportunity to grow.

Don't be afraid or embarrassed to use your nose. That's why we have senses. The only way to tell if you are getting a decent melon, nectarine, peach, or pineapple is to let your nose search for the scent of sweetness and ripeness. Scent translates into taste. Experience is the teacher here. If you are new to shopping, expect to make mistakes, but by paying attention you can avoid a great many.

Avoid any vegetables or fruits that are moldy, shriveled, bruised, or slimy. The idea here is not simply to make certain that food is safe, but that it tastes good, and the freshest, healthiest produce will be safer. Although freshness itself is not a guarantee against contamination, pathogenic organisms will grow more rapidly on decaying produce. Bagged salads and prepared vegetables are a convenience, but make sure the vegetables inside show no sign of age. If the cut edges are brown, discolored, or dry looking, or if there is too much water in the package, do not buy it. Spoilage is a sign that the product has had time for microorganisms—both good and bad—to multiply.

Because fresh fruits and vegetables are perishable, buy only what you need or expect to eat in the next few days. Some seem to have been made virtually permanent these days, perhaps with genetic engineering or irradiation. Plants that haven't been tampered with deteriorate quite quickly. There are exceptions, of course. Carrots, potatoes, onions, rutabagas, and winter squash store nicely for long periods of time. That's the way our ancestors got through the winter. You do need cool, dark conditions, however, for proper storage of root vegetables.

Treat produce kindly. When you are shopping, put it in the top of the cart to avoid bruising—a bruise is an engraved invitation to a microbe. You may think it a waste to use the plastic bags provided, but better some waste than to put your vegetables down on a conveyor belt at the checkout counter that has just had chicken or hamburger drip across it, or to have it touched by a checkout person who has been handling meat products, some leaking from their cartons, off and on all day. Either one is a potential source of contamination.

Wash all produce before you consume it. As the spokesperson of the United Fresh Fruits and Vegetables Association cautions, "Remember, you never buy the first apple you pick up." Many other people have touched the fruits and vegetables you purchase, not only as they were being picked or packed, but in the open bins of the grocery store. Potatoes and carrots were once sold at the grocery store with visible dirt clinging to them—after all, both are root vegetables that grow in the ground. Today they have been prewashed and seem clean. But wash them again. Even wash fruits and vegetables that have a tough skin, such as melon. Cutting with a knife will carry any bacteria onto the interior surfaces, and if left unrefrigerated the microbes could multiply. Cut cantaloupe caused a *Salmonella* outbreak in just such a way.

What about convenience vegetables? Those open boxes of seemingly clean, mixed salad greens and those handy sacks of cut-up, prewashed, salad-ready vegetables? Remember Haylee Bernstein and the other 21 people who became ill from *E. coli* O157:H7 on baby lettuce greens. The question you need to ask is, Who washed these, where, and in what? Chances are, you won't be able to find out, but if the water was contaminated, the lettuce or chopped cabbage will be too. If you must have your convenience, wash these products well before you serve them, remembering there are never any guarantees, just opportunities to reduce your risk. (And if you figure out how much you're paying for someone else to do the cutting, and you may want to do it yourself.)

Don't let produce get overheated in a closed car. Put your vegetables and fruits away promptly. Most do better in the refrigerator, and the crisper has a slightly higher humidity. All cut vegetables and fruits need to be refrigerated. Some whole fruits can be left out of the refrigerator. They get eaten more frequently if they are in plain sight. Salad greens can be washed, spun dry, and kept in a plastic bag, ready to use, but most vegetables will keep better if washed just prior to cooking—especially berries, which spoil quickly if they are prewashed.

How can you be sure your vegetables are really clean? Well, you can't, not with a scientific degree of certainty. But recent studies do show that washing can truly help. Some experts say to wash produce under running water. That doesn't mean a quick swipe under a running tap. Keep a separate plastic tub—white is good for seeing dirt—for washing vegetables. Fill it, then dunk and swish all leafy greens several times. Repeat the process until the water remains clear. Scrub carrots and potatoes and their like individually and thoroughly with a stiff brush. A natural-bristle brush is best as it does less damage; plastic can be brutal. For more delicate produce, such as cucumbers, use a bit of an olive-oil-based kitchen soap, then rinse thoroughly. (I have found both the soap in bar form and these brushes in good kitchen-supply stores.) The produce marketing individuals can tell me from now until forever that the waxes (often containing a fungicide) that are applied to vegetables are safe, and I will still wish they weren't there. They really can't be removed except by peeling, but at least the greasy feeling of some of these vegetables can be reduced. If you look and ask, you can find vegetables that haven't been waxed. The waxing is there to extend shelf life and thereby increase profits for distributors. (If enough shoppers rebelled at buying waxed produce, it would soon disappear.)

There are companies that produce solutions for washing vegetables. The USDA says they work, if used precisely according to instructions. South American women routinely use a bit of vinegar in the vegetable wash water. Many microbes dislike an acid environment. In fact, recent studies have demonstrated that vinegar in one spray bottle and hydrogen peroxide in another can, if sprayed one after the other, kill microbes. Some people, who want more of a guarantee, use a chlorine bleach solution. If you do this, measure carefully and don't overdo it, as chlorine bleach comes with its own problems. One teaspoon to a quart of water is enough. But the spokesperson for the United Fresh Fruits and Vegetables Association says their group does not recommend it. She says they try hard to keep chemicals off fruits and vegetables and don't fancy consumers adding their own. (I personally wouldn't consider using chlorine on anything I planned to eat.)

The outbreaks from fruits and vegetables, although worrying, have not been so frequent that we have to become "paranoid." In fact, we hear about them precisely because they are unusual. Having said that, there is one worry that isn't going away anytime soon. Too many outbreaks have occurred from sprouts of various types. Grown in a moist and warm environment from seeds (recent studies show that *E. coli* O157:H7 is especially adapted to surviving under the dry conditions on seeds), the process is ideal for growing microbes as well. At a recent conference at the CDC, an investigator told of inoculating sprouts with a culture of bacteria and finding it both on the outside of the sprouts and within the stem. The FDA now recommends that children, the elderly, and anyone with a compromised immune system abandon eating raw sprouts.

Remember, heat will kill all these bacterial contaminants, so cooking any fresh vegetable thoroughly will render it safe from these microbes.

Buying good produce is not a casual matter. To get the very best requires knowing something about how and where the product is grown, what its seasons are, and what it should look like at its best. You should also know how long it will keep, how to store it, and how to use it. The manager of your produce counter, your greengrocer (if you are lucky enough to have one you probably live in a major city), or your farm-stand vendor can tell you a lot. Books available at the local library and information on the Web, from such sources as the Produce Marketing Association, can tell you more. There is a lot to learn, but the benefits make it worthwhile.

MEAT

Assume that all raw meat is contaminated with bacteria. Some kinds are harmless. Others are pathogenic and must be avoided. Bacteria get onto meat when it comes in contact, often during slaughtering or processing, with animal waste, whether fecal material or ingesta (material from the animal's upper digestive tract). This should not happen. Ritual slaughter practices, whether kosher or halaal (prepared according to Muslim food standards), are designed to avoid this contamination, and ordinary, nonritual slaughtering plants try to prevent it as well, but still it happens, even in the best of situations. The good news is that all the harmful bacteria on meat can be destroyed by thorough cooking. The bad news is that meat can, if not handled with care, contaminate other foods. This means that the hands, utensils, in fact anything that touches meat or meat juices can carry bacteria to the next thing it comes in contact with. When you understand this completely, preparing meat becomes an exercise fraught with danger. Imagine this: A mother is preparing hamburgers and her toddler drops something out of the high chair. Without thinking she leans over, picks it up with her contaminated hands, and in giving it back also hands her child a potentially fatal dose of *E. coli* O157:H7 or another pathogenic microbe.

The scenario is no exaggeration. In one case of infection from this microbe, two teenagers came in after school and prepared hamburger patties, one after the other. Both cooked their burgers well done, but one became ill. It happened like this. The first boy cooked his burger. The second one placed a raw burger in a pan with a cake turner as the first boy's burger was ready to be taken from the heat. The first boy then used the cake turner to pick up his cooked hamburger. He was the boy who became ill, presumably from contamination transferred to the cooked burger from the raw burger. Knowing stories like this can make you a nervous cook where raw meat is concerned.

Meat safety begins at the grocery store. Have all your meat put in separate plastic bags so that the juices, which contain pathogenic microbes, don't spill onto other food products, then put all the meat in one separate bag.

Store meats in the coldest part of the refrigerator. Plan to use raw meats promptly. Don't allow juices to run down onto foods meant to be eaten raw or without recooking. Think of these juices as poison. If they leak onto refrigerator shelves, wash them thoroughly with hot, soapy water or a germ-killing solution.

Hamburger—in fact, any ground meat product—is a tricky issue. When meat has contamination on the outside, grinding will spread it throughout the product. The most contaminated meat product on grocery store shelves, according to USDA baseline studies, is ground turkey, which many consider a healthy choice. Hamburger meat is first ground not at your local store, unless you are extremely fortunate, but somewhere in Iowa, Colorado, Nebraska, or elsewhere from a hundred or more cows from several different countries. Then the coarse ground meat is packaged in "chubs," long 10-pound packages. The industry considers that it can stay unfrozen for 18 days before it is sold. It is reground at the local retail facility, where more meat scraps may be added. Nothing about this product appeals to me. Mass production means that one contaminated animal can taint 16 tons of hamburger meat. Fresh doesn't mean 18 days old. Adding more meat scraps at the local level further complicates matters.

Your store may be the exception. You may get fresh ground meat. But when you ask if the hamburger is freshly ground, and the answer is yes, you have to ask a second question: "Did you get it in coarse ground?" If the answer is yes, I would suggest finding an alternative. Many Jewish friends tell me they remember their grandmothers buying meat and grinding it at home. This is certainly safer. The chances of that one piece of meat being contaminated are very much lower, and one can at least be certain that the hamburger is fresh. (This technique is no guarantee for poultry, as virtually all poultry is contaminated when it comes from the store, either with *Campylobacter* or *Salmonella*.) Most people wouldn't consider taking the time to grind meat at home today, and the question is, Why not? If you're worth a slightly more expensive hair dye, as a television ad used to tell us, then surely you and your family are worth the extra time and money to eat a safer hamburger product. The other safe choice is to avoid hamburger (which is what I do).

Whatever the source, ground meat must be prepared carefully. Steak tartare is now the equivalent of Russian roulette, and eating a rare hamburger is taking a dreadful and unnecessary chance. If you want thrills, try hang gliding.

Hamburger—indeed, all ground meat—needs careful handling and thorough cooking. A meat thermometer should read 165°F to ensure safety. If you don't have a thermometer, then steam is a good indication of doneness. Brown color is no longer considered a sign of doneness as there is something called "premature browning," which may occur before the meat reaches a safe temperature, but under no circumstances should a child eat a pink hamburger.

A word of caution on using a thermometer. Remember, if it is not handled and cleaned properly, it can transfer bacteria from a raw to a cooked product. Wash it thoroughly before reinserting it if you are testing a food. The USDA has pages of information on their web site on what types of thermometers are appropriate and precisely how to use them (see the appendix). The very complexity is profoundly off-putting. Far better to simply clean up the meat before it reaches the consumer.

But thorough cooking isn't enough. Wash your hands carefully before and after preparing raw meats. Indeed, wash them before putting anything into your mouth. Keep separate cutting boards for meats and vegetables and don't interchange them. Plastic was always thought to be safer on the assumption that the product wouldn't absorb the microbes. Now it seems that the cellulose molecules in wood actually absorb and kill microorganisms, while with plastic they sit on the surface where they can form biofilms that are difficult to remove, even with scrubbing. Either kind is fine if you wash them thoroughly in soap and hot water after use and allow them to air dry. Long ago, watching the kitchen cleanup in a fine French restaurant, I saw the kitchen help carefully rubbing down the wooden cutting surfaces with salt at the end of the evening. This sounds like a good idea for large butcher blocks that can't be moved to the sink. Most microorganisms don't like a heavy dose of salt.

Before preparing meat, remember to have all the utensils and pans that you plan to use out on the counter so that you won't have to open a drawer or cupboard with your contaminated hands in midprocess. If you are cooking on the grill and carry burgers or other raw meat products out on a platter, remember to bring a clean platter for the cooked meats. Putting them on the platter the raw meat was on will recontaminate them.

Muscle meat is sterile, so the good news is that if you don't poke or pierce a piece of meat such as a steak, and you do cook it thoroughly on the outside, you can have it pink on the inside. But take care. One outbreak of *E. coli* O157:H7 occurred when roast beef was cooked rare after having been skewered to cook rotisserie style. The skewer had carried the contamination to the center of the meat, where it had not received enough cooking to destroy the bacteria.

Cook all chicken or other poultry thoroughly to avoid *Salmonella* or *Campylobacter* infection. Cook all pork thoroughly to avoid both the parasite that causes trichinosis and the bacterium *Yersinia entercolitica*. When barbecuing or using a marinade, do not apply the sauce throughout the cooking process or at the end. If the meat has marinated in the sauce, the sauce will already be contaminated; if the meat hasn't marinated, moving the brush from the uncooked meat to the sauce will effectively contaminate it. The sauce on the meat must cook as thoroughly as the outside meat to be safe. Used marinade sauce applied at the end is an anointing with contamination. Throw it away or reheat it to 165°F before serving it with the meat.

One last but important word about cooking meat in a microwave: Don't. It doesn't cook evenly, and can leave contaminated areas. Even the beef industry no longer recommends it.

FISH

Every bite of fresh ocean fish I eat I consider might be my last—not because it might kill me, but because it is so difficult to get these days. Who has seen a piece of cod, a delicious fish once so common as to be denigrated as "servant food," in the last three years? The scarcity is due to increased demand and overfishing. In fact, if consumers knew the truth about the fishing industry— the dreadful waste of what is known as "by catch," the less-than-desirable fish and sea life also caught in nets that are shoveled back into the water, dead and dying—the outrage might keep them from buying fish at all. Interestingly, scarcity can have a direct impact on health. Is your fish fresh? There are things you should know.

Once the advice for buyers was that fresh fish had no fishy smell. I was never sure what this meant. All the fish I had ever eaten had a fishy smell, albeit mild, until the boys across the road brought me a piece of striped sea bass they had just caught and cleaned. There was absolutely no smell, and I realized with a shock that I had never before cooked such truly fresh fish. The taste, which was incredible, confirmed that impression. The only way to get fish this fresh is to know the fisherman, and if you really love good fish, that's an option. The explanation for the scarcity is our dwindling marine resources. Scarcity means a fishing trip is no longer a day trip for fishermen along the Massachusetts and Maine coast and, I presume, elsewhere. Instead fishermen go out for a week or more at a time. Fish are packed in ice in the hold and form strata of progressive layers of freshness, with the freshest being the uppermost layer. Restaurants know this, and the best of the restaurant buyers have arrangements to get these fish when the boat comes in. The best restaurants even have spies up and down the coast scouting good fish, which is why ordinary mortals have a tough time of it. Buyers for specialty shops probably get the next layer. I'm not sure who gets the bottom layer, but to judge from some of the fish I'm offered (but don't buy), I think it might be some of the places I shop.

Buying fish is once again a job for the senses. First, make sure the fish is presented on a bed of fresh—not melting—ice. The bellies should be down. Don't buy any cooked seafood displayed on the same ice, as it may have become contaminated.

If you frequent the fish counter often enough, you can begin to tell from the way a piece of fish looks whether it is old or not. If the fish is whole, the eyes should be clear and bulge a little. (Walleye has naturally cloudy eyes.) There is a fresh "look" that is a mixture of tension, a certain gloss, moisture, and smell. If the flesh doesn't spring back when pressed, the fish isn't fresh. If you see darkening around the edges of the fish or brown or yellow discoloration, it isn't fresh. Don't be afraid to use your senses—that's what we have them for. And don't be embarrassed to ask to check out the fish at close range. It's your money and your stomach.

You don't have to depend on your senses entirely. I rely a good deal on my fish merchant. Trust is important. If someone knows you as a regular picky customer, you will be respected and are unlikely to be told a "fish story." (If you are and find the fish spoiled when you get home, take it back.) One of my approaches is simply to ask which is the freshest and best fish available. Given that responsibility, the person behind the counter is likely to give you a straight answer. If you have a predetermined preference that day and see the fish offered, ask when it came in and where it came from. Ask if it was previously frozen. Of course, that's not good enough. I really want to know what stretch of water it came from, who caught it and when, and a thousand other bits of information. I want the life history of my fish. But that's unrealistic. I settle for what I can learn, which is better than accepting without question what is offered. At the very least, you will begin to establish a reputation as a customer who is not to be trifled with. If the fish you went to the store for isn't up to standard, be adaptable. Pick something else.

Salmon today is generally farm-raised and may have been fed antibiotics from time to time. No connection has yet been made between farm-raising and pathogenic microbes that affect humans, but the interaction of crowded conditions, lack of diversity, and antibiotic use may in the future have an effect. The cheapness of shrimp is also credited to worldwide shrimp-farming operations. There are numerous concerns about these "farms" and their environmental impact, and some expect an eventual repercussion on human health. One word of warning: Frozen shrimp have been cooked, but they also have been handled. It would be wise to recook them to avoid the possibility of microbial contamination.

You may wonder if you are safe buying any fish. It is a good question if you don't live close to the sea and even, sometimes, when you do, although new regulations apply modern safety concepts to fish. Theoretically it should now be possible to trace a fish back to its source, in case of an outbreak (which is too late for the victims, of course). Buy seafood in season—yes, it does have a season—for the best and the freshest. Learn what is seasonal in your area and exploit that freshness.

Still, one hears dark tales of less-than-fresh fish and scallops being rinsed in chlorine bleach water to freshen them up. If you detect any chlorine odor, don't buy the product. The same goes for an ammonia odor.

Obviously fresh fish is critical if you eat sushi, assuming you have found a restaurant and a sushi preparer you trust. These restaurants must find the freshest and highest-quality fish possible to stay in business. Still, always be on alert. One hears that the best, most knowledgeable, and exacting customers get the choicest fish. It's always so, I'm afraid. Customers have to build their own reputations. Also, don't prepare sushi at home.

Frozen fish is an alternative for people who do not live near a source of good seafood. It does not taste as good, because the process allows the cells to leak fluid, so it may be dry and won't have much flavor. However, in many cases it is frozen right on the ship that caught it and could be the safest alternative if you don't live near water. Don't buy frozen seafood if the package is broken, torn, or crushed on the edges or if there is any sign of frost, ice crystals, or pooled frozen liquid, which could be a sign of thawing and refreezing.

Shellfish fall into a category all their own. Most, in fact nearly all, illnesses related to seafood come from shellfish, generally when they are eaten raw or lightly cooked. If you have any kinds of health problems, strictly avoid raw shellfish. Remember, many wonderful dishes use shellfish that are thoroughly cooked. Thorough cooking will kill most of the microbes, although not the toxins from algae blooms. However, oystermen know to avoid these, and mussels are now mainly farm-raised for the commercial market. If you do insist on eating raw shellfish, it becomes not just a luxury but a necessity to know exactly where it came from—some waters are definitely cleaner than others. This can be a challenge. At a famous regional oyster fest some of the oysters served were actually flown in for the occasion; those oysters caused an outbreak of illness. You must ask, and hope you're getting a truthful answer. Don't assume.

Shellfish can sometimes be gathered or dug. Check that it is legal and make sure the place you have chosen is not affected by a poisonous algae bloom.

The old advice to eat shellfish only in months with an R simply means to avoid shellfish in the summer months when the water is warm and conducive to microbial growth. That advice becomes more and more sensible as pollution of beds increasingly becomes a sad fact of modern life. But the nice thing about not eating something out of season is the pleasant anticipation that comes from waiting for it. This is a concept that needs reviving, not simply because it has implications for food safety, but because it makes life more fun.

Recommended Cooking Methods for Safe Oysters Use These Guidelines Provided by the FDA:

- Live oysters in the shell should be boiled for 3 to 5 minutes after the shells open. Boil them in small amounts, as those in the center may not be thoroughly cooked. Throw out any that don't open.
- Steam live oysters 4 to 9 minutes in a steamer that's already steaming.
- Shucked oysters must be boiled for 3 minutes until the edges curl, or fried in oil for 3 minutes at 375°F, or broiled 3 inches from the heat for 3 minutes. Baking in a dish will take 10 minutes at 450°F.

Since raw fish or shellfish has the same potential to harbor pathogenic microbes as any other raw animal product, it must be treated with the same care in the kitchen to avoid cross-contamination.

EGGS

The present situation, in which every egg must be considered potentially contaminated, is, in my opinion, a tragedy. People who don't cook may not realize this, but the potential contamination of the egg by *Salmonella enteritidis (SE)* from the inside out means that breakfast classics—soft-cooked eggs in any form: boiled, poached, coddled, soft-scrambled, sunny-side-up, and over-easy—are now things of the past if one wants to avoid the risk of infection from this pathogen. More worrying still is the number of classic dessert and luncheon dishes that this turn of events affects. In one classic French cookbook 80 percent of the recipes using eggs would now be considered very risky by food-safety specialists. This represents an enormous loss in cultural and culinary diversity, and as a trade-off for cheaper eggs and higher profits for the egg industry it is totally unacceptable. Food lovers everywhere should rise up and proclaim their anger and their refusal to accept this state of affairs. Pasteurized eggs will not do. Dried egg white is not an acceptable substitute. We must have our safe, fresh eggs back. In the meantime, those of us in the kitchen have to accept reality and deal with the hand we've been dealt. (Stay angry, however.)

Once it was only cracked eggs that had to be avoided; the crack could allow the pathogen entry. They should still be avoided. But now that the bacterium can get inside a hen's ovary, eggs have the potential to come prepackaged with *Salmonella*. If that weren't enough, the thorough washing in warm water that eggs now receive creates conditions in which they may be exposed to more contamination (the washing removes the protective coating on the outside of the shell), and the water can spread contamination around. Then the warmth of the wash water heats up the contents of the egg, and slow cooling in the cardboard carton effectively creates the appropriate conditions for microbial growth. Traveling from producer to distributor to retailer, the eggs may not be fresh and may not be refrigerated along the way. Egg dating is written in a mysterious code (often using the number of days in the year—101 means April 1), and television exposés have discovered instances where eggs have been returned to the distributor and then repackaged.

This serious situation with eggs is a fairly recent development, and you can be forgiven for thinking that you have always eaten poached eggs and never gotten sick. Now you might. The *SE* outbreaks began in England in the early 1980s. By the mid-1980s the bug was causing outbreaks in the New England area. Now every part of the country has experienced them. In fact, instances of *SE* have now been reported virtually around the world.

When *SE* was first noticed, quick action such as rigorous, regular testing and sanitation requirements, diverting eggs from *SE*-positive plants to pasteurization, refrigeration requirements, or even destroying contaminated flocks might have stopped the problem. None was implemented on a regular basis. Until very recently, consumers were not even warned of the risks of undercooked eggs. (In fact, the public is being blamed for "undercooking" eggs without being told that the way they had been preparing them for centuries had suddenly become unacceptable because of the appearance of a new and dangerous pathogen.) The egg industry lobbied intensively and successfully against USDA efforts to control this pathogen. (This story is told in detail in my first book, *Spoiled*). Now the industry is stuck having to face the fact that, according to the USDA, 650,000 cases of egg-related *Salmonella* are taking place every year in the United States, causing 650 deaths. The egg industry continues to say that only 1 out of 20,000 eggs is contaminated. The two sets of numbers don't make sense. The second is more likely to be wrong. In any case, getting rid of *SE* will be much more costly and much more difficult than it would have been earlier.

What this means for the consumer is that eggs must be treated like raw meat—as if they were contaminated. To be safe, avoid all dishes that call for anything less than thorough cooking of eggs. Tests done preparing fried and scrambled eggs under laboratory conditions with inoculated eggs found that only hard scrambling at high heat killed *Salmonella;* all other methods left bacteria. The USDA recommends cooking eggs until the yolk and whites are firm, not runny, and have reached 160°F.

Do not allow children to lick batter containing raw eggs or to eat homemade raw cookie dough. (Commercial cookie dough from the cooler section of your supermarket is made with pasteurized eggs.) Avoid cross-contamination by making certain that liquid egg doesn't drip or smear on food-preparation surfaces. Wash your hands well after breaking eggs. Blenders are a special problem as egg can get down in the crevices and be difficult to remove. Pathogens can grow in those crevices. Clean them thoroughly, or better yet, don't mix raw eggs in the blender.

Eggs are perishable; buy only the amount needed for one or two weeks at a time. They should be kept refrigerated at 40°F or below. If you take eggs out of the refrigerator, do not leave them out for more than two hours. Don't use cracked eggs, but neither should you wash commercial eggs as they have already been washed. In fact, you can leave them in the container. Don't store them in the door as it may not be cold enough. The USDA advises that you use raw shell eggs within five weeks (although this seems excessive to me, given that they may have been stored before you bought them) and hardcooked eggs (in the shell or peeled) within one week.

Cooked eggs should be eaten at once and served hot. They can be refrigerated for several days. If you prepare something with un-cooked or lightly cooked eggs that is to be cooked further later, re-frigerate it immediately until final preparation.

Recommended Cooking Times for Safe Eggs

Scrambled eggs Cook 1 minute at 250°F (medium-high heat).

Poached eggs Cook 5 minutes in boiling water.

Hard-cooked eggs Cook 7 minutes in boiling water.

Sunny-side eggs Cook 7 minutes at 250°F (medium-high heat) or covered for 4 minutes at 250°F (medium-high heat).

Fried and over-easy eggs Cook 3 minutes at 250°F (medium-high heat) on one side, then 2 minutes on the other side.

For dishes made with eggs Bring egg temperatures to 160°F, and follow these guidelines:

> **Sauces or custards** Cook until the mixture coats a metal spoon.
>
> **Quiches and egg-based casseroles** Bake until a knife comes out clean.
>
> **Meringue** Bake at 350°F for at least 15 minutes.

Now that widespread contamination is a fait accompli, the egg industry is offering some interesting advice as to how traditional dishes can be prepared. It's apparently not impossible, but it does take time and effort.

To cook egg whites before adding them to a mousse or a cold soufflé, they must be combined with the sugar in the recipe. Use at least two tablespoons of sugar per white. Cook the mixture over low heat in a heavy saucepan or double boiler. Beat as you cook until the whites stand in soft peaks. The sugar keeps the whites from simply coagulating. (Do not add cream of tartar if using an alu-minum pan or the mixture will turn gray.)

To cook egg yolks, you need another liquid in a ratio of two tablespoons of liquid per yolk. Less and you get scrambled eggs. Cook very slowly in a heavy pan, stirring constantly until the mixture coats a metal spoon, bubbles at the edges, or reaches 160°F. Cool quickly and include this mixture in the recipe. Meringue pies are difficult to cook safely, but it can be done, the egg industry says. A three-egg-white pie meringue would take 15 minutes at 350°F and should reach 160°F. More eggs will take 25 to 30 minutes at 325°F. Flaming meringue to achieve a browned look does not cook it sufficiently to be safe. Refrigerate properly cooked meringue pies.

The alternative is to use liquid pasteurized eggs or dried egg whites. Having to resort to these products is distressing. Their use should be resisted unless you have no other option.

There is, fortunately, one more choice for those within shopping distance of Massachusetts. Eggs produced and sold by The Country Hen in Hubbardston, Massachusetts, are from hens that have never tested positive for SE. They are also fed organic grains and are not kept in cages. These eggs are worth every penny you have to pay for them, which is about twice as much as ordinary eggs. They can be used when you want to take what has become a "walk on the wild side," and prepare an old favorite like Caesar salad. Check to see if there is an egg producer—it will probably be a smaller one—that applies the same standards and does the same testing near you. If there isn't, but word gets out that these are popular eggs, there soon will be. But typically the industry is looking for end-point technological fixes such as pasteurizing eggs while still in the shell. Don't settle for these options. The only real solution is to establish a goal of naturally clean fresh eggs and to do whatever is necessary to achieve it. Of course, consumers must expect to pay more.

PROCESSED FOODS

It is a cruel irony that some of the safest foods are also the most thoroughly processed. The techniques of canning foods are such that what is inside is sterilized and also protected by the can from further contamination (although one would like to know if the can was seamed with lead, which California has a law against). That many of these foods have lost some of their nutrition and a great deal of their taste in the process is simply a fact of life.

Commercial cake and cookie mixes are prepared with pasteurized eggs, and unless you add a fresh one the batter won't be harmful. Cereals were a pretty safe bet until the 1998 outbreak from cereal contaminated with *Salmonella agona*. Now there seems to be no guarantees, although that outbreak can be considered a rarity. Still, if you want guarantees, there's oatmeal or other cooked cereals.

Generations past were warned to avoid dented or swollen cans, and this is information that should be revived. Even a small dent can create microscopic holes, allowing contamination to enter a can, and a swollen can is a sign that bacteria inside have survived the time in the retort and begun to reproduce. There have been outbreaks from canned foods, but they have been rare. Today a system is in place in the United States that helps to ensure safe canned products.

Frozen foods also go through processes that make them less likely to be contaminated, although there have been notable exceptions, such as the cases of cholera in Baltimore in 1991 linked to frozen coconut juice from Thailand. There have been outbreaks from ice cream, but hopefully the unfortunate experience of one producer was a warning to others to make sure their premix is free of contamination.

Treat frozen foods carefully. At the grocery store put them together in a single bag. Take them home and promptly put them into the freezer. Do not refreeze foods, but if you have left something out and it still contains ice crystals and is very cold to the touch, it should be alright to put back in the freezer, and it is certainly safe to eat at once. Frozen foods will keep safely virtually indefinitely, but quality—taste and texture—is an issue. Frozen storage of three to four months is about average for ham or corned beef, six to twelve months for steaks, one month for bacon, three to four months for TV dinners, two to three months for soups and stews, a year for whole chicken or turkey, but only nine months for poultry parts. Frozen leftovers last about two to three months. Egg whites can be frozen for a year. Deli and vacuum-packed products, mayonnaise, prestuffed products, and store-prepared salads, to name a few, don't freeze successfully.

Thawing frozen foods should be done in the refrigerator or the microwave. For example, when a turkey is left to thaw on the counter, the outside won't stay cold enough to prevent the growth of bacteria. Plan ahead. A 20- to 25-pound turkey will take five days to defrost in the fridge. Even an 8- to 12-pound turkey will take one to two days. A guide for turkey or large pieces of meat: Figure 24 hours for every five pounds in a refrigerator set at 40°F. If you push it to the back where it's colder, it could take longer. Also, a glass shelf will keep the turkey colder than a wire shelf. Probably needless to say, the Food Safety and Consumer Education Office of the USDA's Food Safety and Inspection Service doesn't advise thawing the turkey on the back porch or the car trunk where its progress can't be monitored. However, I must admit that where I live in Maine my uninsulated back porch has on occasion become a short-term refrigerator. Use common sense, and monitor the temperature with a thermometer that records high and low if possible.

You can also thaw frozen poultry in cold water, allowing 30 minutes per pound. Thaw it in a leak-proof plastic bag to prevent contamination and water absorption. Immerse it, checking from time to time to be sure the water is cold. If you thaw poultry in a microwave, be sure to cook it at once, as some areas may be partially cooked in the process, and bacteria could reproduce.

PREPARED FOODS

One has to be more concerned today with prepared foods sold at deli counters or prepackaged on the cooler shelves. Both have grown in popularity in the last 20 years as people with busy lives discovered how convenient, if more expensive, it is to buy foods prepared by others. One of the biggest problems is *Listeria,* since it can grow under refrigeration. The outcome for pregnant women can be so profound—the infection can cause miscarriage and fetal abnormalities and has a 25 to 70 percent fatality rate—that pregnant women should absolutely avoid the deli counter. Soft cheeses, uncooked hot dogs, cold precooked chicken: All of these have been implicated in outbreaks. Recalls of foods such as hummus and potato salad happen too often—there were more than a dozen recalls for *Listeria* in 1998. And 1999 proved to be a banner year for the pathogen. A single outbreak killed 13 people and one recall of contaminated luncheon meats and hot dogs followed another. Convenience comes at a price, and it may be higher than previously suspected. These are foods easily prepared at home, where the risk of contamination can be controlled.

It is also important to remember that prepared foods are perishable. Sometimes prepared and prepackaged fresh foods are treated to avoid the obvious signs of spoilage, but it is spoilage that indicates that other microbes, which may give no sign of their presence, have had a chance to multiply. Using organic acids or replacing oxygen in bags of vegetables with other inert gasses to hold down spoilage bacteria may be helpful for the food processor but a bad idea for the consumer.

Pay close attention to "use by" dates on prepared foods. They may be conservative, but when it comes to food safety, you should be too. Discard any product with mold or any other sign of spoilage. Do not used luncheon meats that have a slippery feel, look iridescent, or show any other signs of spoilage. When in doubt, throw it out. It's never worth taking a chance.

Proper storage of leftovers is very important. How many families leave the Thanksgiving turkey sitting out after dinner? It can brew up a fantastic growth of pathogenic microbes, as many people have discovered to their dismay. It's a better idea to cook the stuffing separately from the bird and to promptly refrigerate both at the end of the meal. Thoroughly cooked sliced turkey can last for a week or more when refrigerated. Never leave cooked foods out of the fridge for more than two hours. To be completely safe, cooked foods should be thoroughly reheated to 165°F or until steam is visible.

THE CLEAN KITCHEN

There are a number of different strategies for maintaining a clean kitchen. One approach is to eat out. But for those of us who actually cook and eat, it's more of a challenge. It is not possible to establish completely hygienic conditions in a real family-kitchen environment, but every improvement translates into safer eating. (Those of you who already keep perfectly clean kitchens need not read this section. This is very elementary information, but if you need it, you know who you are.)

A philosophical perspective needs to be established at the onset. Mind-sets matter. Accept the fact that safe food and cleanliness are linked and are important. Food needs a clean, appropriate place to be stored, whether it is the refrigerator or the pantry. Begin there.

Prepare yourself with cleaning materials—sponges, old rags, buckets, soap, or a cleaning solution of your choice—and proper food wraps. Foil, plastic wrap, and even waxed paper are handy; containers that seal are helpful as well. These can be inexpensive plastic freezer containers, recycled plastic containers from yogurt or cottage cheese (carefully cleaned, of course), or glass containers with either glass or plastic lids. Jars can also be recycled as storage containers.

Drawers should be cleaned and lined. Lining that can be wiped is handy but expensive. Something as inexpensive as recycled wrapping paper or paper bags will do just as well.

Begin with cupboards or the fridge. Attack one thing at a time. Take everything out. Get rid of old food, leaking bottles, questionable items, bits of moldy cheese, and so forth. Give the interior a complete scrubbing with a suitable cleaning substance and a sponge. Baking soda works well. Even simple hot, soapy water will do fine. If you really want to disinfect the surface, use either the bacterial solutions on the market or a tablespoon of chlorine in a quart of water (slightly more than one would use to wash vegetables). There are less toxic alternatives at health-food stores.

Get in the cracks and crevices where microbes lurk. Take out the vegetable crispers in the fridge and other removable parts and clean behind them. Give that ketchup bottle a wash under the tap to be sure what you put back is clean. Wrap up the cheese in foil—it will keep better.

Begin thinking about containers for virtually everything. Loose dry foods, such as rice, flour, beans, and other grains will keep better and evade infestation from bugs and rodents if they are kept in sealed containers. Glass canning jars from France with clamp lids are wonderful things. They are expensive but last virtually forever. Nuts, raisins, and anything else small and prone to becoming rancid or spoiled that keeps better under refrigeration can go into saved jars.

Glass refrigerator containers for leftovers can still be found with a little effort.

Think about getting an old-fashioned bread box. Bread doesn't really need to be kept in the fridge, but it does need a safe place. Bread boxes that can be scalded from time to time with boiling water, as grandmother did, are still available.

One of the nastiest items in the kitchen is the blade of the can opener. If yours is electric, ask yourself why. A good manual can opener (not the cheap metal versions on sale at the grocery store but a sturdy, efficient model with a good solid crank) is easier to use and can be popped into the dishwasher or manually washed after each use.

Sponges can get very nasty. Putting them in the microwave for a minute will cook the microbes out. Rinsing them out with a germ-killing soap is helpful. In fact, just washing them carefully after use can't hurt. Paper towels are highly recommended because you throw them away, but what an enormous waste. Consider old-fashioned dishrags and tea towels that can be popped into the washing machine frequently. Sponges can be put in the wash as well. When you are conscious of the potential to spread bacteria around—especially if you are, say, wiping up meat juices—you'll begin to keep your sponges cleaner. Understanding microbes does that to a person.

Unpack groceries as soon as you get home, and put away and store everything properly. Eggs and milk need to be kept cold. Don't put eggs in the door—its not cold enough. Be sure that meats are not put where they can drip on foods meant to be eaten raw, or where they can drip on anything. Cold cuts need to be kept cold and separated as well from foods meant to be eaten raw. Oils, once opened, can go rancid. Some, like olive oil, become thick and difficult to use after being refrigerated. A good solution is to keep on the counter a small amount in a dark bottle (light degrades the product) to be refilled from time to time.

The many disinfectants and antibacterial products that have been rushed to the market in response to new fears about foodborne disease raise concerns of their own. Microbiologists wonder if using products designed, for instance, particularly for *Staphylococcus* might actually create an ideal environment for other pathogens. In fact, the liberal use of antibacterial products may do exactly what antibiotics have done and create resistant bugs. They aren't necessary if basic tenets of cleanliness and food safety are followed. Hot water and detergents or soaps are very effective.

Basic common sense and thoughtfulness apply. One solution: If you are worried about the pathogens that meat brings into your kitchen, don't bring meat into your kitchen. This is what I have done, and I worry a lot less about the state of my kitchen counters—which, when all is said and done, is a good thing.

4

Surviving Foodborne Disease as an Adult

The signs of foodborne disease are usually, but not always, unmistakable. Most commonly, one or more of the following occurs: nausea, vomiting, diarrhea, fever, lethargy, and cramps. (Just to make things confusing, these could be symptoms of something other than foodborne disease.) On the other hand, the first symptoms of infection with *C. botulinum* are dizziness and trouble with vision, speech, and breathing. Fish toxins can produce symptoms ranging from nausea and diarrhea to tingling, itching, flushing, and numbness in the extremities. And infections with foodborne pathogens can have unexpected repercussions from symptoms that seem unrelated.

Nevertheless, you are likely to know all too well that you are ill. Your doctor may not, however, be able to identify the cause because the symptoms frequently mimic other ailments. Often the intense cramping of *E. coli* O157:H7 has led physicians to mistake the infection for appendicitis or intussusception of the bowel (what one physician described as the bowel rolling in on itself like a sock). Unnecessary surgeries are performed quite often when the cause is actually a pathogenic microbe.

While certain rare infections may manifest themselves through unusual symptoms, the garden variety vomiting–diarrhea–cramping illness calls for the same basic treatment. Forget most of what you think you know or what other people may have told you. Avoid that initial impulse to rush to the drugstore for diarrhea medication.

Says the World Health Organization (WHO), "Antidiarrheal preparations, including antimotility drugs, can provide an adult with symptomatic relief; however, they can also cause undesirable side effects and an authoritative opinion should be sought before they are used. They should never be used by children."

What are diarrhea medications, and are they ever called for? The National Institutes of Health looked into the matter with regard to travelers diarrhea. Looking at what are called "adsorbents" to reduce loose stools, they found activated charcoal to be ineffective. Kaolin and pectin, which are widely used ingredients, give the stool more consistency but reduce neither the cramps nor the frequency of the episodes, nor was the course of infectious diarrhea shortened. Doses of bismuth subsalicylate preparation at a rate of one ounce every 30 minutes for eight doses was also found to lower the rate of episodes by one-half, although this difference wasn't seen in the first four hours.

They report no studies that support the effectiveness of *Lactobacillus* preparations or yogurt, but that may be because no drug companies want to do them. Anecdotal reports, long experience in Europe, and common sense in understanding the theory of "competitive exclusion," whereby the gut is reinforced with "good bacteria," would lead one to try this method, since no harm as been attributed to it. As dairy products are generally not advised for diarrhea sufferers, "probiotics" such as *Lactobacillus acidophilus* in capsule form can be found in health-food stores. AIDS patients subject to chronic diarrhea have anecdotally reported good results.

There are other diarrhea medications called "antimotility agents." Some are natural opiates, such as paregoric. Loperamide and diphenoxylate bring quick symptomatic but temporary relief. They should never be used in patients with high fever or with blood in the stool, and they should not be used if symptoms last longer than two days. And as the WHO points out, they should not be used by children.

There seems to be different advice coming from the WHO and the National Institutes of Health (NIH). While the WHO really discourages treatment with commercial antidiarrheal medications, the NIH implies they have their uses. Be your own guide, but take note that U.S. advisers often seem to favor the interests of commercial producers more than does the WHO. Despite a request from the WHO to prohibit all sales of diarrhea medication for children, the United States has refused to do so.

It's well to remember that the body knows what it's doing when it's in a diarrhea mode: It is ridding itself of something that shouldn't be there. Certainly with a vicious pathogen like *E. coli* O157:H7, one would want to get rid of it as soon as possible. The greatest danger to the body, whatever the cause of unrelenting diarrhea or vomiting, is dehydration. Fluids must be maintained.

The goal of proper treatment is to avoid dehydration. If the diarrhea is mild and sporadic, dehydration probably won't be a problem. But dehydration can quickly become so if you are having four to six stools a day. In severe cases, with 10 or more stools a day, it *will* be a problem if you are not *very* careful.

In the case of mild diarrhea, chicken broth or diluted fruit juices are suitable for replenishing fluids. Small, frequent meals are best, and some say to avoid extremes of hot or cold foods. Avoid drinks with caffeine or alcohol, fatty foods, irritating spicy foods, and dairy products.

If the diarrhea becomes more intense, it is very important to pay close attention to your own condition and to drink appropriate liquids. Avoid anything too sweet, such as soft drinks or even sports drinks. There are much better choices than plain water, which diarrhea experts say is not absorbed into your system as it travels too quickly through the digestive track. Instead, keep at hand, whether you are at home or traveling, packets of oral rehydration solution made to the WHO formula. These are not easy to get (see the appendix for sources). The commercial packets of hydration maintenance salts available in most drugstores are made to suit the tastes of children, and they are better than nothing, but the formula is too sweet for maximum effectiveness. It is possible to make up a simple solution that is effective (see p. 183 for a recipe). Sip the fluid slowly and try to get down two to three quarts a day if you are an average-size adult. The following is the exact WHO formula, for those with precise scales and the inclination to search for the ingredients, which may be available at your local pharmacy:

For one liter of clean drinking water (boiled and cooled before mixing if there is any doubt):

3.5 grams sodium chloride
2.9 grams trisodium citrate dihydrate (or 2.5 grams sodium
bicarbonate)
1.5 grams potassium chloride
20 grams glucose (or 40 grams sucrose)

Studies in Baltimore and other cities have shown that oral rehy-dration therapy is a cheaper, simpler, and more effective alternative to hospital care. Estimates are that a nationwide savings of $500 million is possible if oral rehydration solution (ORS) were more commonly used to avoid expensive intravenous rehydration. One qualifier: If the diarrhea is bloody, fluids still should be maintained, but ORS is not a suitable treatment.

Diarrhea experts have found that it is very important to maintain a nourishing diet during a diarrheal illness. This means continuing a good intake of carbohydrates and protein, if possible, and still avoid-ing fats, dairy products, and spicy foods. It can be a challenge if the diarrhea is accompanied with vomiting, but crackers or dry toast are traditional foods to eat slowly when you are at your worst and hav-ing trouble keeping anything down. You can progress to chicken broth with rice or noodles, and plain cooked rice. Bananas are a good source of potassium, which you will be needing, as are boiled potatoes. A little steamed fish would be a good choice for some first protein as you begin to feel better. Gradually add cooked vegetables. If nothing else can be kept down, rice water can be prepared by cooking rice with a much larger proportion of water than usual and drinking the liquid left in the pan when the rice is soft.

The signs of dehydration to watch for are a cessation of urination and an increasing lack of tension in the skin. There will often be a pronounced thirst. The mucous membranes will be dry. Dehydrated skin, when pinched, will hold its shape for a moment. With severe dehydration the skin may actually stay tented for longer, the eyes may seem sunken, the extremities may feel cold, and obvious signs of confusion may appear.

Confusion and what people have described as "a kind of crazi-ness" that can manifest itself in irrational behavior constitute the truly unfortunate aspect of severe dehydration. A Baltimore woman ill with cholera reported that she reached the point, after prolonged, persistent diarrhea, when she knew she was acting strangely and knew she needed fluids, but she simply no longer cared. When she was taken to the hospital she was found to be severely dehydrated. Dehydration can lead to death; it is a very serious matter. In cholera epidemics it is dehydration that kills, and it can do so very quickly, sometimes within a matter of hours. Thus it is important that a partner, spouse, parent, or caregiver be equally aware of the need to maintain appropriate fluids and to recognize the signs of dehydration.

Most diarrheal illnesses are self-resolving, meaning you will get over it yourself in all likelihood. There are some signs, however, that should send you to the doctor. If there are indications of severe dehydration, go to the emergency room. If the diarrhea continues for more than three days or if blood is in the stool, see a doctor. The CDC recommends that all bloody stools be cultured for *E. coli* O157:H7, which is now a reportable infection almost everywhere in the United States.

Your physician will probably look for signs of dehydration and may take a stool sample to culture or examine for parasites. In the prevailing atmosphere of cost-cutting medicine, culturing is not encouraged by some HMOs or health plans because diarrheal illnesses usually go away by themselves. But if your illness is quite severe, a stool culture or examination will help your physician decide how to treat it. In some cases an antibiotic is appropriate; in most cases it is not. It could well make things worse. Only identifying the culprit can determine that for sure, although other symptoms may give a physician a good idea of whether an antibiotic is needed. How long has the diarrhea gone on? Does it wax and wane? Parasites and viruses have patterns of infection that differ from infections caused by bacteria. A physician can make an educated guess that the lab needs to look specifically for parasites, or he or she may ask the lab to look generally for both. Because the tests are difficult and expensive, only rarely will a physician look for viruses, but viral gastroenteritis is usually short-lived in any case. It's also important to remember that diarrhea can have other causes—many other causes—and those need to be eliminated as well.

Recent studies have indicated that most doctors are unaware of exactly which pathogens laboratories routinely check for, and different laboratories may have different standards. Only gradually have many begun to regularly look for *E. coli* O157:H7 when there is a report of bloody stools, and even today the use of the particular culture medium most suitable for finding this pathogen is not universal. Some labs still do not routinely look for *Campylobacter,* even though it is the most common cause of diarrheal disease in the United States. In view of this, it is a good idea to ask your physician exactly which microbes the stool is being cultured for, and if your stool is bloody, ask particularly that O157 be looked for. The answer as to what the lab routinely tests for may surprise your physician, but at least he or she will no longer be making unwarranted assumptions.

There is another reason why it is in everyone's interest that stool cultures be undertaken more often. If a laboratory spots a number of cases of diarrhea from the same pathogen—or better yet, subtypes it and finds a number of illnesses from an identical strain—there is probably an outbreak under way, probably related to a single experience or a single food. Discovering what is causing the illnesses, especially if it is a mass-produced, widely distributed food, can trigger an investigation and perhaps a recall, thus preventing other cases. Or it might, even if the outbreak is over, further medicine's understanding of the pathogen and what foods it can be found in. It will certainly give a better overall indication of the numbers of cases caused by particular pathogens. So while there may be a short-term economic advantage to avoiding the expense of culturing stools, there is a considerable long-term advantage to the community at large in doing these tests. In a perfect world public health concerns would trump private healthcare profits.

What if the physician reports that your stool culture has come back negative? Does it mean that you don't have a foodborne disease? It could. It could also mean any of the following: the pathogen had already left your body; the culture was performed incorrectly; the pathogen was so sensitive that it didn't survive transport; the laboratory didn't look for the particular microbe that was causing the problem; or the illness was not foodborne. In short, a negative stool culture simply means a negative stool culture. It means that the physician cannot be sure what was causing the illness. If he or she has not waited for the stool culture and has prescribed an antibiotic, the chance of discovering the cause is further decreased.

It would be nice to think that physicians are all up to speed on foodborne diseases, but from reports of people who have sought treatment, it seems clear that information is inconsistent and varies from excellent to dismal. Health-care professionals often refer, confusingly, to "stomach flu" as "going around" when there is really no such thing as stomach flu and "going around" gives a misleading view of how diarrheal diseases are transmitted—somehow implying that they are inevitable and that nothing can be done to prevent them. If they are "going around," keep in mind it is through fecal contamination, whether of contaminated food or water, or from person to person or from person to food. These are not infections you pick up from taking a deep breath in a movie theater. Careful hand washing and care about what goes into your mouth can limit the transfer of diarrheal disease.

Medical personnel often ask the wrong questions as well, such as, What did you have for dinner last night? Most of these pathogens take longer than a few hours to cause illness, anywhere from one to 14 days, depending on the culprit. Without an investigation or an ongoing outbreak from a specific pathogen with highly defined symptoms of infection, such as *Cyclospora,* it is almost pointless to speculate on the cause. The exception would be when several people who normally don't see each other have dinner together and several days later all get sick. If you are curious, you can speculate on that kind of common denominator. But if you are part of a couple, you both are sick, and you eat together every night, it's probably wrong to point to last night's restaurant dinner as the source of your misery. It could just as easily have been the hamburger you prepared at home two or three nights before.

Finally, health-care workers sometimes give the wrong advice about how to treat foodborne disease. Automatically prescribing an antibiotic without a clue to the cause is not a good idea (although again, there may be reasons it is appropriate, but ask the physician why), nor is simply providing the advice to keep up fluids or suggesting the consumption of ginger ale or sports drinks to prevent dehydration. They probably won't hurt if the diarrhea is mild, but they won't help much, and if there is any sign of dehydration they may be very ill advised. A proper ORS is the best solution for non-bloody infectious diarrhea.

One last thought. One person in a household with foodborne disease is more than enough. If possible, have that person use a bath-room separate from the rest of the family. Be certain that it is disin-fected with either a commercial product or a tablespoon of chlorine bleach in a quart of water. Wash soiled towels and sheets in disinfec-tant as well. Good hand washing and careful food preparation are also important. In this way an illness can often be contained. It can be much more serious if passed on to a very young child or an older person. Deaths have occurred from just such person-to-person transfer.

5

Children and Foodborne Disease

It would be perfectly possible to begin this section with a horror story, or even several—stories of infants and young children who have been exposed to foodborne pathogens through food, or from person-to-person contact, or in swimming pools, and who have become seriously ill and died. Such scenarios are among every parent's worst fears, and the news media have toyed with those emotions all too frequently, perhaps until many parents have simply tuned out from anxiety. There is certainly reason to worry. Children are more susceptible to foodborne infection than adults because their immune systems are immature, and the younger they are, the greater the risk. Foodborne pathogens are certainly present in the food supply and in the environment, but having said that, concerns about children must be put in perspective.

This story is not only more typical than the horror tales, it is funny. A couple, the wife a well-known author and the husband a photographer, were both vegetarians. In the interest of letting their son make up his own mind about his diet, they encouraged him to try many foods, and at least when they were eating out, to eat meat if he felt inclined. He had always taken his lunch to school, however. One day he decided to branch out and, in the spirit of adventure, eat the cafeteria lunch. You can guess the rest. It was the day virtually everyone who ate in the cafeteria ended up violently sick from a foodborne infection. The illnesses were mild and over quickly, and everyone recovered completely, but what an introduction to the wider world of food!

The best and safest way to nourish an infant under a year is to breast-feed, whether at home or traveling. Additionally, an infant less than a year old should not be given honey, because of the danger of infant botulism. For other recommendations about infant feeding, consult your pediatrician. But infants are just as susceptible to person-to-person transfer of infection as anyone else. Frequent hand washing is vital for the parent or caregiver, especially before feeding the infant.

You can be very careful about what your children eat at home; you can be careful about hand washing; you can be certain your kitchen is clean; but when your child leaves the house, whether to day-care, school, or a friend's home, or in any public setting, you lose a degree of control. In a sense that's part of being a parent and part of a child's development. A parent who knows what dangers lurk out there can become paralyzed with fear. The best defense is to know and understand the basics of how these pathogens work, to be thoroughly familiar with how they are transmitted and which foods, environments, or activities are likely to put a child at risk. Then you can take reasonable, commonsense precautions.

Increasingly families with two working parents must resort to day-care for their children. It may be best to look upon them as toughening facilities for youngsters, because they will be exposed to any illness in the neighborhood. The vast majority of children survive the experience. A mother told me her first child, who did not attend day-care, got all the same infections as the younger child who did, but just got them later when he entered kindergarten. Nevertheless, there are some especially virulent bugs you don't want to expose your children to. Children have been infected with *E. coli* O157:H7 at day-care and nursery schools. One of the four children who died in the 1993 Jack in the Box outbreak was infected not by a hamburger but at day-care from another child made ill from a hamburger. In another *E. coli* O157:H7 outbreak in a day-care facility, the source was the wall-to-wall carpet that had become contaminated by a child with diarrhea. I personally consider carpeting a real hazard in day-care facilities. It doesn't take a genius or a scientific study to realize that it simply cannot be thoroughly cleaned, and children are in constant contact with what could well be a contaminated surface. It is, however, virtually ubiquitous. It will take a revolution to get rid of it.

Children who attend day-care facilities are clearly at more risk from diarrheal diseases than children who are cared for at home. What is often not considered is that their families are as well, because they bring the infection into the family environment where, if parents are not careful, it can spread from one member to another. During an outbreak of giardiasis 25 percent of family members of infected children also had the infection. In an outbreak of shigellosis it was found that children attending day-care centers were significantly more likely than other preschool children to be the cause of the illness within the family.

Day-care facilities present special problems, because sick children who probably should be at home, but whose parents can't take time off, spread disease. When an ill child is present, the possible routes of person-to-person transmission are many. Toys, toilet facilities, hands—all can become contaminated and can pass on the infection. The problem of what to do with sick children is a serious one for a parent and the day-care staff as well. If the facility bars the sick child, a desperate parent might simply take the child elsewhere, possibly spreading the infection. A better solution—and parents should suggest and work for this—is to have a separate sick room that has its own bathroom. Unfortunately this is not always practical or even possible in a small facility. Children with a negative stool culture, if the problem has been diarrhea, can return to the main room. Naturally all caregivers should have good training about hand washing, being especially careful after changing diapers or providing toilet assistance and before serving food.

It would be nice to think that children were in the best and safest hands when they start school, but they may not be—or more accurately, the foods the cafeteria serves may not be free of contamination. An *E. coli* O157:H7 outbreak in a junior high school originated with precooked hamburger patties; in another institution for children hamburger meat arrived contaminated. In 1997 parents across the country began to worry when the media pounced on a story about hepatitis A in strawberries distributed for school lunches. Parents perceived it as a new problem, yet outbreaks occur frequently in schools. Many are never investigated.

Other risks at school come from field trips to farms. Children should be told never to drink unpasteurized farm milk under any circumstances. Neither should they drink unpasteurized apple cider. Both have caused illnesses on field trips. Even just a visit to a farm can involve exposure to unfamiliar pathogens simply from petting farm animals, but these trips shouldn't be avoided or ended when thorough hand washing after contact with animals or their environment and before eating is the simple and effective answer to the problem.

It does seem that protecting our children becomes more of a challenge all the time as new or unfamiliar pathogens appear in unexpected places. Most people are aware of the outbreak of *E. coli* O157:H7 infection in Atlanta, Georgia, in the summer of 1998, when children were infected from exposure to water at a swimming facility contaminated by a child with diarrhea. Tragically, one child died. The outbreak was not unique; infections have been traced to contaminated swimming water before.

This brings back memories for some people of long ago, of summers when children swam until the first case of polio was reported in town and then life changed. No swimming in public pools, no visiting fairs or theaters or other places where large numbers of people congregated; even going to church came to a halt. My grandmother, who had read *The Jungle* by Upton Sinclair, a novel about the meatpacking industry, never let me eat hot dogs or indeed any food sold at a carnival. Infectious disease was a looming threat, and avoiding infection became an accepted way of life. There was a lovely interim of about 30 years when infectious diseases did not seem so important. Now they are back with a vengeance, and we need to adjust our lives accordingly.

I personally would never take a young child to a pool where there were children in diapers. I believe that children in diapers should not be allowed in public pools. Such a restriction wouldn't eliminate the risk—adults can be sick and can transmit their infections as well—but it would lower it. (Chlorination of pools *should* solve the problem, but it can be spotty and doesn't seem to be the guarantee it once was.) Decisions of this kind are up to individuals, but they should be well-informed individuals.

Children are so vulnerable when they are away from home. They trust adults to care for them and to provide them with safe food. That trust can be misplaced. Is the parent of your child's best friend attuned to safe-food habits? One of the best ways to give your children a margin of protection against foodborne disease is to teach them, as soon as they are able to follow instructions, not to put their hands in their mouth, and to wash their hands with soap before eating or handling food and after using the bathroom. The second practice takes a lot of supervision. We all probably remember the cursory job of hand washing we did as children. When the towel has dirty finger marks or the soap is still dry, the hand washing wasn't good enough. In the end your child will learn from watching you. Hand washing should become such a habit that it becomes virtually unthinkable for either you or your child to eat or prepare foods with unwashed hands. (If your child reaches this point, be sure to carry hand-cleaning wipes to avoid hysterics on a picnic, in the car, or at some other location without hand-washing facilities.)

Children should also be taught to reject a pink hamburger, undercooked chicken, or soft-cooked eggs no matter who gives it to them. They can point out the undercooking politely and ask that it be recooked; hopefully they will be listened to. A child needs confidence to do this, and that should be instilled as well. It is a vitally important lesson, on a par with not accepting rides from strangers. A child should be taught to turn down invitations to lick the cake bowl or to sample homemade cookie dough at a friend's house. (Commercial cookie dough uses pasteurized egg yolks and is not a problem.) You might also advise your child not to eat from commercial salad bars and to select cooked foods whenever possible. You may think this puts too heavy a burden on your child or is unnecessarily cautious. Again, this is an individual decision depending on how vulnerable you think your child is to foodborne infection.

While children can develop immunity to certain pathogens, some are far too dangerous to be complacent about, and new microbes evolve or appear to which no one has immunity. Two farm children became seriously ill with *Salmonella typhimurium* DT104, a strain resistant to several antibiotics, after drinking unpasteurized milk, which had been their habit from birth. This new bacterium had entered the farm environment somehow, perhaps in an imported calf. On another farm a small child, playing in the hay on the barn floor as her mother milked, developed infection with *E. coli* O157:H7. However fortunate it is to develop immunity, it is not an option to expose children to pathogens to determine which survive and which do not.

The same food-safety tips that apply to adults apply equally well to children—only more so, as they are more vulnerable. Foods served in school cafeterias are generally very safe. If you are concerned about what your child is eating at school, by all means pack his or her lunch and admonish him or her not to eat foods from other sources, remembering from your own school days the temptation to trade lunches.

As serious a problem as foodborne disease is, it is best to put it in perspective. There are so many things to worry about with children, and this is just one more. Plus there are no guarantees to be had. Maintain good habits in your kitchen, model good practices and an attitude of care, and teach your children good habits of eating and food preparation, then relax and enjoy life. Being careful doesn't mean being "paranoid."

Treating the sick child is not dissimilar from treating the sick adult. The difference is that the infant or young child cannot describe precisely how he or she feels, and the parent or caregiver must be alert for signs of severe illness or dehydration.

Here is a typical scenario. Your two-year-old has seemed under the weather, not quite herself. She has an episode of vomiting, followed shortly by diarrhea. The attacks of diarrhea are repeated several times during the day. You try to make her comfortable, but there is something else you should be doing. By supplying a steady supply of *appropriate* liquids, all the while keeping your child eating certain foods and bypassing other foods, you can almost certainly avoid complications that could be very dangerous.

There are 1.5 billion episodes of diarrhea per year in children around the world. The World Health Organization (WHO) says that four million of these end in death. Most of these cases occur in underdeveloped countries where sanitation may not be good, and living conditions may be difficult. Yet diarrhea is still one of the most common illnesses in children in the United States, where the Centers for Disease Control and Prevention (CDC) estimates that each youngster will experience seven to 15 episodes by the age of five. While it is usually self-resolving, it can also be severe enough to require hospitalization. In fact, nearly 10 percent of hospitalizations in the United States of children less than five years old are associated with diarrhea, and 300 to 500 children die each year after a bout of diarrheal disease. Some who recover from serious infections may be left with permanent consequences. Children are equally, if not more, susceptible to some of the complications and chronic aftereffects of diarrhea.

Experts at the WHO and the CDC believe these numbers for hospitalizations and deaths could be brought down significantly if diarrhea were properly treated at home with a program of maintenance and oral rehydration therapy (ORT) using an oral rehydration solution (ORS). Ironically, this method has been used around the world, especially in underdeveloped countries, with great success for 25 years; some credit it with saving more than a million lives a year. The development of this simple and inexpensive method of restoring body fluids and electrolyte balance is uniformly seen as one of the great medical achievements of the 20th century precisely because it has saved so many lives and is available at a cost that virtually anyone can manage. An expert in treating diarrheal disease tells a story of missionaries to Uganda who took along an oral rehydration mix for their own use. When they saw local individuals too weak to stand because of diarrhea, they mixed their powder with water and used it as directed and within hours saw these victims literally back on their feet. "Resurrection fluid," they called it.

Nevertheless, ORT is virtually unknown and certainly very underused in the United States and Canada, where one specialist admits that rather than *prevent* dehydration, some doctors favor waiting until a child is dehydrated, then hospitalizing him or her for IV rehydration, *then* releasing the child with instructions to maintain fluids. Various organizations that support ORT use say it is reluctance on the part of physicians, a reluctance that appears to be based on outdated studies and misunderstandings coupled with cultural bias, that is stalling more widespread use of ORT in North America.

One can only guess at the reasons for this reluctance. The treatment, while extremely effective, is low-tech in the extreme; a package of premeasured and mixed powders is mixed with clean or boiled water and administered slowly to the ill child. It may well be that American medical consumers feel more comfortable with high-tech medical procedures, despite the inherent dangers of complication from invasive treatments, such as IV rehydration. Another possible reason may be taste. The mixture, at the ratio of salts favored by the WHO, has an unappealing salty taste that children may at first refuse.

Perhaps the chief reason is that early tests with ORT some 25 years ago had the occasional adverse side effect of hypernatremia (too much salt in the blood) when the solution was mixed and used improperly. Since then the mixture has been modified for maximum efficacy, and while a small danger remains that the patient will get too much salt, it can be easily avoided if parents or caregivers are given good instructions and follow them exactly. If parents in the challenging conditions of the least-developed countries can be trained and trusted to use the treatment effectively, there is no reason that parents in the developed world cannot do the same.

The CDC, in its report on treating children with acute diarrhea, says quite bluntly, without reservation, "The combination of oral rehydration and early nutritional support guides a patient through an episode of diarrhea safely and effectively. When the principles of therapy that are outlined are accepted by all levels of the U.S. medical community, and when education of parents includes instructions about how to begin ORT at home, than unnecessary hospitalizations and deaths can be prevented."

It is past time to take an aggressive approach to training mothers and other caregivers in the proper use of oral rehydration therapy. The packets, which keep for three years or longer in temperatures less than 85°F, should be in everyone's medicine cabinet, and anyone who takes care of a child should be familiar with ORT.

Serious hurdles must be overcome. Many physicians are unaware of the latest studies on ORT's effectiveness—especially when combined with an effective feeding program—and some assume that effectiveness in developing countries has no application here. Thus many clinicians, to judge only by what mothers say, continue to prescribe a variety of "clear liquids" to treat diarrhea. Some of these, such as ginger ale or other clear sodas, may, because of their high sugar content, make the diarrhea worse and actually lead to an imbalance in electrolytes.

Giving plain water is counterproductive as well, because it goes through the system too quickly to be absorbed. It is not enough, as some mothers have confidently told me, simply to "keep the fluids, any fluids, flowing." It is the critical mixture of salts and sugars that makes absorption easier, and to be most effective, the ratio of sodium, potassium, citrate, and glucose is essential. Often the BRAT diet (banana, rice, applesauce, and toast) is recommended. Most experts now say this does not have enough nutritional content and does little for dehydration.

There is one more reason the developed world often opts for expensive hospital intravenous rehydration. (It costs nearly 10 times as much to treat dehydration with an intravenous drip in a hospital as it does to administer ORS, according to a UNICEF publication.) Treating a child with the oral rehydration solution takes time. It may mean patiently feeding the liquid by spoonful or dropper. Rehydrating intravenously is faster and more efficient from a certain standpoint, but it carries with it inherent dangers (from infection, for instance). If our busy lives can't include the appropriate treatment of a sick child, we have to ask ourselves exactly what our values and priorities are.

What is absolutely clear is that parents in developed countries need to get the same kind of training that mothers in third-world countries get about how to guard against dehydration in their children, how to prepare and give oral rehydration solution, how to maintain proper nutrition, and how to recognize the signs of dehydration in their children that indicate a need for immediate medical care.

There are over-the-counter rehydration therapies available in a solution. They are usually not made to the formula that WHO testing has found most effective, but they do help *prevent* dehydration.

What is causing your child's diarrhea? Rotavirus, for which there is now a vaccine, and which is apparently not foodborne, has been the single most common cause of diarrhea among children, responsible for one-quarter of the cases worldwide, but it is less common in the United States, where the cause can also be other viruses (Norwalk-like and other caliciviruses, enteric adenoviruses, astroviruses), bacteria (*Salmonella, Shigella, Yersinia, Campylobacter,* various strains of *E. coli, Vibrio cholera*), or parasites *(Giardia, Cryptosporidium, Entamoeba histolytica)*. Many of these pathogens are food- or waterborne. Oral rehydration works effectively for acute and watery diarrhea, no matter which of these pathogens is responsible. (Persistent diarrhea, lasting two weeks or more, or bloody diarrhea is a different matter and will be discussed later.) What you should *not* do is give your child an over-the-counter diarrhea medication.

According to the *WHO,* "Antidiarrheal drugs should never be used [to treat children with diarrhea]. None has any proven value and some are dangerous." The CDC concurs, saying, "Little evidence exists to support the use of nonspecific drug therapy in children, and much information exists to the contrary." The WHO called for a ban on certain preparations and at least 10 developing countries as well as several developed countries have complied. The United States has not. One drug that is particularly dangerous is diphenoxylate hydrochloride with atropine sulfate (Lomotil and other brand names, available by prescription). In 1991, 30,000 prescriptions of liquid diphenoxylate were filled in U.S. retail pharmacies, mainly for pediatric use. My local pharmacist says he has received no prescriptions for its use in children recently, and that seems good news. The packaging of commercial preparations of loperamide hydrochloride—Imodium, Imodium A-D, Pepto Diarrhea Control, and others, available by prescription and over the counter—generally indicates that the drug should not be used in children less than 12 years of age. These warnings should be adhered to.

It seems only common sense, but while diarrhea may be the sign that a microbial invader is attacking the body, it is also the way the body gets rid of something that is upsetting it. It is therefore counterproductive to stop the process artificially. Still, a child on the simple ORT may continue to have diarrhea, even while avoiding dehydration. This continuing diarrhea often leads the mother to abandon the ORS, which would be a mistake. Feeding starchy foods, such as rice and potato, and avoiding fats and sugars can help bring it to an end. (CeraLyte contains rice in the mix and has been shown to be effective in decreasing stool volume, as has Ricelyte, which contains a glucose obtained from rice.)

When is ORS not recommended?

- Bloody diarrhea
- Severe dehydration
- Prolonged diarrhea—over two weeks (A parasite may be involved in this case.)
- Intractable vomiting (although if the ORS is given every one to two minutes by the spoonful it will help). Do not allow a thirsty child to drink large volumes of ORS fluids.

When should you take your child to the doctor?

- Bloody diarrhea: A child with bloody diarrhea should see a physician, who should request a stool culture, specifically asking, in addition to the usual search for culprits, for tests for *E. coli* O157:H7, which requires a special culture medium and may not be routine.
- Prolonged diarrhea: Diarrhea that goes on two weeks or more
- When mild dehydration is not corrected or when there is any sign of acute dehydration

How can you recognize dehydration in your child?

Dehydration is a serious condition that may be avoided with careful and early home care for diarrhea and vomiting. The parent or caregiver of an infant or child is the first clearinghouse for illness in the child. It is therefore important that caregivers learn the basic signs of dehydration. They are quite easy to spot, even to the nonprofessional eye. The younger the child, the more apt he or she is to dehydrate, because infants and young children have a higher body-surface-to-weight ratio and a higher metabolism, and they are dependent on others for fluid (being unable either to ask or to turn on the tap by themselves). Any sudden weight loss is a good indication of dehydration, but other signs include slightly dry mucous membranes, watery diarrhea, and a decreased urine output. A pronounced thirstiness may be the first sign of mild dehydration.

Indications of moderate dehydration include, along with an increase in those symptoms, a loss of skin tension (when it is pinched, for instance, it may stay "tented" for a second) and sunken eyes. In infants there may be a depressed fontanel.

Severe dehydration must be treated at once in an acute-care facility. Signs are severe lethargy or an altered state of consciousness; the skin, when pinched, may take as long as two seconds to return to normal; the feet and hands may feel cold, due to poor circulation; and there may be rapid, deep breathing. In an infant, a lack of urine output for 12 hours should be a sign of concern. Go to the emergency room.

What are commercial oral rehydration salts and where can they be found?

There are a number of products on the market made especially for treating diarrhea in children. None of them has the ratio of salts that the WHO or the CDC recommends, although they can be useful in *maintaining hydration* in a child who is not yet dehydrated. Shockingly, the packets of mixture that cost pennies in underdeveloped countries sell for $1.50 or more per packet (I paid $6.24 for a package of four packets of Kaolectrolyte), 10 times what they cost in the third world. I paid $6.59 for a liter (a quart and 1.8 fluid ounces) of Pedialyte, a similar but ready-mixed solution that is even further off the ratio recommended by the WHO for rehydration, although it says clearly that it is a "maintenance solution" rather than a rehydration solution. But expert analysis says these products will, if used as directed, keep a child from becoming dehydrated.

Another popular brand of electrolyte replenisher is Ricelyte, which one study has shown to be successful in both rehydration and maintenance, even though it too is not manufactured to the WHO standards. (Other products that resemble the WHO standards to varying degrees and are available in Canada include Rapolyte and

Rehydralyte for rehydration, and Gastrolyte and Lytren for maintenance.) CeraLyte is produced to WHO standards, and while seldom available in U.S. pharmacies, may be obtained from the company or from a catalog specializing in medical supplies for travelers. Simple WHO-standard oral rehydration salts can also be obtained from a company in Kansas City that packages them in traveler 20-packs, which may be more than any parent needs to have on hand, but could be divided among several parents. This is the most cost-effective way for Americans to purchase the packages unless one belongs to a co-op and buys them by a case.

Presumably taste is a factor, and the WHO mix is not particularly pleasant. Once children expected medicine to taste bad. Now they expect it to taste good, and some parents find it difficult to make their children do anything at all, even when their health depends upon it. Making your child understand that he or she must consume this fluid, that refusing it is not an option, may well be the first step in successful prevention of dehydration at home. If there seems to be no other recourse, Pedialyte also sells ready-to-be-frozen pops containing the maintenance dose, although it doesn't sound like a good idea for a child to think a frozen pop is medicine.

Says the CDC, "Pedialyte, Ricelyte, and other similar low-sodium solutions can be used for rehydration when the alternative is physiologically inappropriate liquids or IV fluids." All these brands advise parents, quite appropriately, to use these fluids rather than juices, soft drinks, sports drinks, or water. The leaflet in Kaolectrolyte is especially helpful. "Avoid fluids that contain a lot of sugar such as soft drinks, undiluted juices, or fruit punch," it says. "These drinks can actually make diarrhea worse." Kaolectrolyte also offers good advise on how to administer ORT, which is by spoonfuls every few minutes. Their advice about continuing to feed the child and their suggestions of good foods and bad foods are equally appropriate and helpful. This product also has a toll-free telephone number for advice. While the packets need to be mixed with water (measuring carefully), they are simple to store, are good for up to three years, and are handy in emergencies. They can be easily carried when traveling.

Pedialyte provides no food advice and suggests that the fluid be used only "under the supervision of a doctor," which defeats part of the purpose, which is to avoid an unnecessary doctor's visit. It also says to "offer" the liquid to the child every three to four hours, instead of every few minutes. Pedialyte has no toll-free number. The premixes have a shorter shelf life than the packages of powder.

What can you do in an emergency?

In an emergency—on a camping trip to the North Woods, perhaps, with no corner drugstore available—you can prepare your own oral rehydration solution. Remember to measure all quantities precisely as even minor deviations from these recipes could be dangerous to your infant.

Starch-based solution	Sugar-based solution
1 quart clean water	1 quart clean water
½ teaspoon table salt	½ teaspoon table salt
2 ounces (about 1 cup) baby rice cereal	8 teaspoons sugar

How much should your child receive?

An infant should receive one liter over 24 hours. A child should take in one liter over eight to 24 hours. For mild dehydration the fluid should be given using a teaspoon, syringe, or medicine dropper, gradually increasing the amount as it is tolerated. If, after two to four hours of this treatment, the patient no longer shows signs of dehydration, the maintenance approach can be taken.

Is there a way to maintain hydration?

According to the CDC, breast-fed infants with diarrhea should continue nursing on demand. For bottle-fed infants, "full-strength, lactose-free, or lactose-reduced formulas should be administered immediately upon rehydration in amounts sufficient to satisfy energy and nutrient requirements." If such formulas aren't available, the full-strength lactose-containing formulas "should be used under supervision to assure that carbohydrate malabsorption doesn't complicate the clinical course." Otherwise, dilute the lactose-containing formula at first, but rapidly restore it to full strength.

An older child can receive semisolid or solid foods. Starches, cereals, yogurt, fruit, and vegetables are appropriate. Avoid foods high in simple sugars and fats.

When fluids with more than 60 mEq/l (milliequivalents per liter) of sodium are used for maintenance, other low-sodium fluids such as breast milk, diluted or undiluted infant formula, or water need to be given as well to prevent sodium overload.

If my child still has diarrhea on the ORS, should I discontinue it or try a commercial over-the-counter product to stop it?

No. The glucose-based ORS restores the body's electrolyte balance, but it does not stop the amount or the duration of diarrhea. Restoring appropriate foods early in the disease episode can reduce the diarrhea.

Should my child receive an antibiotic for diarrhea?

In general, the answer is no. It could make things worse by wiping out the competitive bacteria in the gut that are holding down the intruder. Your physician might consider them when dysentery or high fever is present, when watery diarrhea lasts for more than five days, or when stool cultures, microscopy, or an epidemic indicates a specific cause for which a specific treatment is appropriate.

6

When It Isn't Over

In 1988 Nancy Howard lived with her husband and two children in a rambling 10-room Victorian house on Cape Ann in Massachusetts. Just before the Christmas holidays Nancy invited over members of her extended family and spent the whole day cooking. Looking back, she says she had two bad cooking habits. She tasted both the raw cookie dough and the meatballs as she was preparing them. The dinner went off well, but just before midnight she woke up with severe abdominal pains. "It was incredible pain," she remembers. It passed, and she went back to sleep but soon woke up again with another bout of pain and then fierce diarrhea. Her first thought, every cook's nightmare, was to wonder if she had made everybody sick, but her husband was lying beside her deep in contented sleep.

She definitely wasn't well, however. For the next two days Nancy was in increasing misery. She made it through Christmas Day on her own, but on the 26th she had to call a doctor. She reported that she had no fever, and he advised her that the illness would probably pass and to stay away from milk products. A savvy "doctor" mom, she already knew that. But with no fever, she couldn't convince him of how absolutely awful she felt. She knew she was quite ill, but the doctor—her own was away—was quite dismissive. He told her to call back in 48 hours if she hadn't improved. She did just that, but found that she was so weak she could hardly tell her story. She didn't realize it, but she was probably suffering the effects of dehy-

dration as her diarrhea continued unrelentingly. Nevertheless, she
didn't care for the doctor on duty and waited until her own was
back on call. When she saw him on the 29th, he said at once that
her trouble was likely a bacterial infection and gave her an antibiotic; he also took a stool culture, looking for the usual suspects—
Salmonella, Shigella, and *Vibrio.* At this point Nancy had lost 10 to
12 pounds. Because she was a petite woman, this represented more
than 10 percent of her body weight. She was also still sick—so ill
that she couldn't swallow the antibiotic tablets without vomiting.
Her doctor then gave her a prescription for Compazine, to treat the
vomiting, but by then she was so weak and debilitated that even
getting the prescription filled seemed "like a mountain to climb."
When Nancy did get the medication and managed to get the antibiotic down, she began to feel a little better. By New Year's Eve
she was sipping sports beverage and chicken broth, her unrelenting
diarrhea had begun to slow, and she started to feel as if she might
have a future.

However, her ordeal was not over. She awoke in the middle of
the night with terrible pain and realized her knee was swollen to
the size of a grapefruit. The pain and swelling were so impressive—
she remembers never being in such pain before—she went early on
the morning of New Year's Day to the emergency room of her
local hospital. The physician on duty seemed resentful, perhaps of
being there on a holiday, and even overtly hostile. He kept asking her, even when the answer was a clear no, if she hadn't had a
sports injury. Had she been playing touch football or something?
"No," she answered. "This is something systemic. This is going on
inside of me."

"Are you a nurse?" he asked derisively. He drew a tube of blood
and sent her home. She was extremely uncomfortable.

Nancy has a wide group of friends who had been very supportive during this ordeal. People had offered to look after the children
and had helped in other ways. They felt she needed to get to Boston
to a hospital quickly. In the meantime the emergency room doctor
called back to say that her sedimentation rate (the speed at which
blood cells settle to the bottom of a column of citrated blood, a
technique used to diagnose the progress of various abnormal conditions) was normal. "Good-bye," he said, and she knew he meant it.

That did it. Nancy felt certain something was seriously wrong. She could no longer walk; now both knees were badly swollen and terribly painful. Her husband took her to Massachusetts General Hospital that afternoon.

The first suggestion—which when her local emergency room physician had suggested it sounded, through his hostile tone, like a threat—was that the fluid be drawn out of her knees with a syringe. She let the staff do it, and at once she felt better. The relief lasted a few hours.

Massachusetts General, where she was immediately admitted, is a teaching hospital, and Nancy found herself surrounded by eager young people, seemingly with little supervision, possibly because of the holiday. They were diligent in looking for the cause of her ailment, perhaps too diligent, she remembers. She was subjected to every sort of test they could think of, "as well as lots of probing and prodding." She told them about her recent episode of gastroenteritis, and they carefully noted it on her chart, even mentioning the cookie dough and the raw meat she said she had eaten. She was dehydrated, and after being admitted, she was given IV rehydration and sent for tests, but three days later no one had yet come up with the cause of the pain and swelling. Nancy was profoundly discouraged.

"No one was helping me. I thought, 'I'm going to leave.' "Then she and her husband remembered that they actually knew someone at the hospital, a physician. They tracked down their friend. A gastroenterologist, his presence turned everything around at once, she remembers. And he knew what she had. His diagnosis was reactive arthritis. A small percentage of people infected with some foodborne pathogens can get this severe reaction.

At once Nancy felt more comfortable. She was certain she had the proper diagnosis now. It made sense. She was told that she *would* get better and was more than likely to have no long-term effects from the condition. That was good news. Still, she had been transformed within two weeks from a strong, healthy mother of two into a wheelchair-bound invalid who needed a visiting nurse and help with her children and her household. She felt estranged, even from some of her friends. No one seemed to know anything about reactive arthritis. If she talked about it, they seemed vaguely uncomfortable. She talked to two other woman who had had the same experience, but in general she felt isolated and alone with her seemingly odd illness.

Nancy's recovery was monitored by the arthritis department at Brigham and Women's Hospital. It took trial and error to find the right medication that would reduce the inflammation without side effects, but eventually she watched happily as weekly tests showed her now high sedimentation rate drop as the inflammation retreated.

Nancy spent a month in a wheelchair. Then walking and getting up and down the stairs remained difficult. Within three months she was beginning to feel normal, almost. The following summer, when staying with friends in Ireland, she found she couldn't climb the ladder to a sleeping loft. Full recovery had taken longer than she realized, although it could have taken much longer.

Today, after a decade, she still experiences the residual effects of her bout with reactive arthritis. Her joints ache if she is under stress or gets sick or the weather takes a turn. Otherwise, she feels she has recovered.

Today Nancy is more sympathetic and understanding of the problems of the handicapped, more patient and tolerant of other people's illnesses. Needless to say, perhaps, she is also very cautious about what she eats.

Reactive arthritis is only one of many conditions known as chronic sequelae of foodborne disease. More and more often now, what were previously thought to be chronic ailments are being found to have infectious causes. A perfect example, of course, is stomach ulcers, now understood to be caused by infection with the bacterium *Helicobacter pylori* (which can be foodborne).

James Lindsay of the University of Florida at Gainsville is an expert on these sequelae as they relate to foodborne infections. In addition to reactive arthritis and other forms of arthritic conditions, he lists ankylosing spondylitis, renal disease, cardiac and neurologic disorders, and nutritional and other malabsorptive disorders as possibly associated with infection from foodborne pathogens. The relationship between these infections and these conditions "ranges from convincing to circumstantial," he says. One reason for doubt is a lack of data collection. After all, the pathogen that caused Nancy's illness was never identified, although the circumstantial link was clear. Adding to the uncertainty is that some of the symptoms may overlap with those of a specific pathogen or they may be wide ranging. Sometimes the chronic disease symptoms can appear without any signs of illness, or sequelae can occur even when the immune system has successfully gotten rid of the primary infection. The chronic condition may also be the result of an autoimmune response. This all means that the issue is confounding. Nevertheless, what evidence there is for many of these chronic foodborne-disease-related ailments is pretty good. Experts estimate that they follow between 2 and 3 percent of infections.

Infection with *Salmonella* can lead to septic arthritis when the infection spreads to the area around the joints. This condition can be treated with antibiotics and can often be cleared up if there has not been permanent joint damage. Reactive arthritis, such as Nancy had, can follow infection with *Yersinia enterocolitica, Yersinia pseudotuberculosis, Shigella flexneri, Shigella dysenteriae, Salmonella* spp., *Campylobacter jejuni,* and *Escherichia coli.* A variation called Reiter's syndrome occurs when reactive arthritis appears together with conjunctivitis (inflammation of the eye) and urinary tract infection.

There are other sequelae. Graves' disease, an autoimmune disease, is now suspected of being an after-effect of infection with *Yersinia enterocolitica* serotype O:3, since antibody responses to the bacterium have been found in the blood of Graves' disease sufferers. Severe hypothyroidism can also occur after an infection with *Giardia lamblia,* but treatment with metronidazole can completely eliminate the parasite; regular thyroid hormone absorption in the intestine then returns.

Crohn's disease and ulcerative colitis are often called inflammatory bowel disease. Although the cause is not entirely clear, these chronic inflammatory diseases have been associated with infectious agents such as *Pseudomonas, Mycobacterium, Enterococcus faecalis,* and *E. coli.*

Renal diseases such as hemolytic uremic syndrome (HUS) are now widely linked in the public's mind to infection with *E. coli* O157:H7, but while that is the major cause, infections with *Citrobacter, Campylobacter, Shigella, Salmonella,* and *Yersinia,* as well as other Shiga toxin–producing *E. coli,* have been known to bring it on. While HUS normally occurs in children, the adult version of the syndrome is called thrombotic thrombocytopenic purpura (TTP). Children who weather HUS may be left with any number of problems due to the tissue destruction and organ damage the syndrome produces. Kidney transplants, colostomy, or damage to lungs, heart, eyesight, or brain—they are all-too-common "souvenirs" in HUS survivors.

Guillain-Barré is another syndrome that frequently occurs after an acute gastrointestinal infection. The disease begins with mild sensory disturbances and leads to progressive motor paralysis. A potentially life-threatening condition, it requires immediate medical attention. Meningitis likewise can follow foodborne disease, especially infection with *Campylobacter.*

Some infections of the heart are linked to foodborne pathogens. Both endocarditis and myocarditis with permanent damage to the heart have been associated either directly or indirectly with foodborne disease. People with ankylosing spondylitis linked to enteric pathogens as a trigger have a high incidence of cardiac conduction abnormalities, says James Lindsay, which may follow other arthritis-like illnesses. In fact, there is a possible connection between foodborne infections and atherosclerosis, or hardening of the arteries, but the causes appear to be a complex blend of factors.

Infections with a number of foodborne pathogens such as Enterobacteriaceae, rotavirus, *Amoeba, Cryptosporidium,* and *Giardia* can produce conditions where foods are not properly absorbed and nutrients are lost. Some diarrheal episodes from these causes can become chronic, but even short bouts of diarrhea "may result in subtle changes in immunologic status." The seriousness of the diseases depends mostly on the immune status of the person and may last for several years or for life. "Death due to diarrheal illness in the immunosuppressed and in persons with AIDS is nearly 80 percent. No effective treatment is available," says James Lindsay. Additionally, people with AIDS can experience other chronic conditions such as coughing and low-grade fever following infection with these pathogens. Even in those who are not immunocompromised, some infections with *Campylobacter jejuni, Citrobacter, Enterobacter,* or *Klebsiella* can be followed by diarrhea that lasts months or even years.

According to Lindsay, one area that is little explored is how chronic infection affects human personality. Psychological effects might result from the chronic pain of arthritis, irritable bowel, or chronic diarrhea, which, he says, "would be enough to make anyone temperamental, moody, or depressed." Studies do show a high correlation between chronic toxoplasmosis and several personality changes. The changes were different in men and women.

Lindsay points out that since foodborne diseases are mostly preventable, recognition by the public and the public health community of these chronic after-effects could lead everyone to take foodborne disease more seriously and to take greater care in avoiding infection.

7

Taking Action

Just as the causes of foodborne disease are many, the cure will come from all directions as well. There will be no quick fix. Repairing the damage to the food supply and making sure that good, clean, safe, fresh food is universally available will involve government, science and public health experts, industry, nongovernmental organizations (NGOs), consumer advocates, and, perhaps most of all, consumers themselves. It is the consumer who will pressure the others into action when the effort stalls.

If that sounds cynical, remember that *Salmonella* cases were increasing exponentially and *E. coli* O157:H7 had been identified as a vicious new pathogen in the food supply a decade before the USDA's Food Safety and Inspection Service (FSIS) took an aggressive stance in attacking the problem of food safety. It was the massive Jack in the Box outbreak, with the public's subsequent interest in not poisoning themselves or their children, that in 1993 finally galvanized the agency into belated and sometimes tepid action.

The reason for the inaction was lobbying on the part of the food industry. In fact, during that fateful decade Congress, with a deregulatory agenda, had systematically reduced the funding for meat and food inspection, apparently on the assumption that the people best able to ensure the safety of food were those who had made the 1906 Meat Inspection Act and the Pure Food and Drug Act necessary in the first place.

The problem with handing industry the responsibility of policing itself is simple. There is no obvious incentive for food producers to make certain their products are safe: Bacterial infections that can make humans sick seldom affect the animals, and despite the newspaper accounts of outbreaks where the cause is found, the majority of illnesses in humans are seldom linked to their source. As the recent report of the National Research Council of the Institute of Medicine puts it, "Because it might be difficult to show that one's illness was, in fact, food-related and to trace it to a particular product, the risk of having to pay damages to consumers for harm is probably not a major incentive for food safety."

This report, "Ensuring Safe Food," is one of a number in recent years that have looked at the federal agencies responsible for food safety and found them wanting. The fact is, it's a wonder the tangled system works at all. While the chief responsibilities for food safety fall under the authority of the USDA (mainly raw animal and vegetable products) and the FDA (mainly processed products and fish), actually a dozen agencies have some role in implementing more than 35 statutes. Responsibilities are overlapping and confusing. The USDA's mandate to promote agriculture while attempting to protect the public creates confusion and opens its actions to suspicion. Attempts by the agency to educate the public to the dangers of food contamination must be reconciled with its inspection system that is meant to be a guarantee of safety and quality. The result is legalistic hairsplitting over such issues as whether the microbes that can make you sick and kill you amount to adulterants on meat, which leads to the handy conclusion that pathogenic microbes are natural on raw animal products and it is the consumer's responsibility to avoid them. They are certainly present on and in animals, but the goal of safe slaughter and processing should be to minimize contamination, and it can be done.

The recommendation of the report is that a single food-safety agency should be established. This is elementary. It should be done now. Unfortunately, bills before Congress to do just that have died an early death. It is misguided on the part of agribusiness to think that food safety is not in their best interests. While in the past it may have been difficult to link an outbreak with a specific food product, sophisticated surveillance and testing now makes it more likely and with greater accuracy. DNA testing can determine that a microbe from a sick individual is precisely the same microbe found in a food product. As these techniques are more frequently employed, evading responsibility will be increasingly difficult. Being identified as the source of contaminated food can have devastating consequences for a company, as Hudson Foods, Foodmaker (Jack in the Box's parent company), and Odwalla Juice well know.

How the conflict between promoting agriculture and protecting the public can lead to disaster has been amply demonstrated in Great Britain, where the reluctance of the Ministry of Agriculture, Fishing and Foods (MAFF) to link mad cow disease with potential danger to humans led to a full decade of exposure of the population to a contaminated product. In the end it was the country's beef industry that suffered the consequences after all, consequences that might have been far less severe if action had been taken sooner. Establishing a single independent food-safety agency that could operate without these conflicts became a high priority in the UK, and it is now in the process of being organized. It will be unfortunate if it takes a similar disaster in the United States to make Congress see what should be obvious: that the best way to maintain, or perhaps reestablish, confidence in the safety of U.S. agricultural products is to authorize a separate, efficient, effective, and independent food-safety agency that speaks with one voice.

One thing the U.S. Department of Agriculture, the Council for Agricultural Science and Technology, the World Trade Organization, and any number of other organizations and interests can agree on is how food-safety standards should be set. The standards should be based on science, they say. We live, after all, in an era in which both science and scientists garner enormous respect. Many of us use science as a standard in other aspects of our lives. Why not use science to tell us which foods are safe and which are not?

There is something extraordinarily reassuring about science. It implies a rational and detached evaluation of empirical evidence in a controlled exercise in which emotion and suspect subjective judgments have been eliminated (although one could show that such assumptions are not always true, and that subjective decisions as to what to investigate and how to conduct research enter into the process at every juncture). To question the value of science as the ultimate arbiter of food safety in this sort of atmosphere is thus tantamount to heresy, but the safety of food depends upon doing precisely that. The problem is that science is being misused in this context and may well expose people to danger for longer periods of time simply because it is by nature cautious, conservative, and often very bad at determining the long-term effects of small changes in the complex food supply.

Clearly science plays a vital role in food safety. It can, for example, tell us which microbes are likely to cause trouble in milk, demonstrate that pasteurization can kill the bacteria, design a process to do this in an efficient and effective manner.

It was not always so. For millions of years humans made personal, subjective judgments about the safety of what they ate, and the accumulation of good and bad experiences was incorporated into food rituals and traditions. While mistakes were inevitable and the learning curve painful, our lives depended on these skills. When we forget to trust our senses, when we set aside our instinctive wariness about what we eat, when we become too complacent and accepting, we can easily get into trouble. In one outbreak where the pathogen was in pasteurized chocolate milk, most of those ill reported that the milk tasted funny but they drank it anyway. Relying on science has led us to mistrust our senses.

While there is no substitute for a scientific approach to studying disease-causing organisms and investigating outbreaks, it's important to recognize that all science isn't equal. There is good science, bad science, and bought-and-paid-for science. When the latest study says that soy products are good for you, factor in the additional information—if it is available—that the study was funded by the soy industry. It is not that the information isn't correct, but it should be evaluated with the understanding that you may not be getting all the information from the study, and that had the results been negative, as the tobacco industry has taught us, we are unlikely to have heard of the research at all. The often conflicting information that emerges from research is an additional and sharp reminder that science is a process, not a promise.

But more important to actual consumers, science is not the standard individuals use when making the ultimate decision whether to taste a particular spoonful of food. Often we cannot explain our preferences or dislikes, but the inability to define where they come from and how they evolved doesn't make them invalid. Science might tell us that thoroughly toasted manure is perfectly acceptable and safe as a protein component in our corn flakes or that a cooked fly in our soup presents no danger, but most of us would have to be mighty hungry to buy into the argument. Instead, it is clear that most people make decisions about foods on the basis of appearance, smell, taste, cultural habits and traditions, previous experiences, and a host of other factors—a heady mix of subjective perceptions and preferences. Most of us would think that however irrational our food preferences might appear, and even if they are not guaranteed to protect us from what we cannot see, we nevertheless, have an absolute right to them.

Science is notoriously challenged in predicting the long-term consequences of small changes in diet or in effectively coordinating the synergistic effects of the many different elements in an individual's diet. When Oprah Winfrey taped her now famous program on beef, her audience uttered a collective and unrehearsed gasp of horror when they learned that cows were being fed to cows. Despite that intuitive response, it took science a decade, even in the midst of a devastating epidemic of bovine spongiform encephalopathy, to reach the same conclusion: Feeding cows to cows was a bad idea. During that decade virtually the entire beef-eating population of Great Britain was presumably exposed to a potentially deadly pathogen.

In fact, much of the enthusiasm for the "science standard" is due not to its strength, but to its weakness. Because science can be challenged and rechallenged, and is inherently clumsy in determining precise cause and effect in the complex environment of the human body and its relationship to food, its very slowness actually favors dangerous food.

The scientific standard for food safety is an essential element of global food trade strategy. Its purpose in this context is not to establish the safest food but to prevent a country from establishing "artificial barriers" to trade based merely on a preference or a perception that a food is unsuitable or dangerous. Thus the desire of Europeans to avoid beef raised on hormones, which has had the effect of keeping U.S. beef out of that market, has been successfully challenged. Their intuitive sense that hormones are not helpful or desirable in meat is irrelevant when science is dogma. If hormones cannot be proved by scientific research to be a health danger—and that might take a long time—then Europeans must eat our beef.

The way around this problem, which would be to label the beef as a U.S. product so educated European consumers could choose to avoid it, is also challenged. The ability of consumers to choose what they want to eat, it would seem, is to be sacrificed on the altar of trade policy, with science as the high priest holding the knife. The obvious solution for U.S. producers, to market hormone-free beef both at home and abroad, is greeted without enthusiasm.

So the problem with the science standard is not science itself, but its inherent weaknesses and its flagrant misuse.

This is not the first time that our faith in science has been exploited duplicitously. In the aftermath of the Jack in the Box outbreak, the meat industry touted science-based inspection as the solution to contamination in meat. Again, it had a reassuring sound. The old inspection methods of touch, smell, and visual inspection (organoleptic methods, they are called) were deemed inappropriate in a scientific age. The implication was that microbial testing was necessary in an age when microbes were the problem. Yet even as the meat industry was implying this was the case, they were fighting microbial testing behind the scenes. What they wanted was their own version of a system called HACCP (pronounced Ha-sip): hazard analysis and critical control points. This approach identifies potential points of contamination, and systems are put into place to reduce or control contamination at those points. This is a scientifically based system. It is a good system when used in certain situations.

Here's how it works in a sardine plant. There is a point—in the retort—when pathogenic microbes can be cooked out of the contents of the can. Record the length of time and the temperature of the can in the retort and you have a safety record that can be confirmed. The accountability, in the form of the company name, is on the can. The problem for raw meat is that (1) there are no points in the process where contamination can be eliminated with certainty and (2) there is no accountability—a package of hamburger doesn't tell you who slaughtered the cow.

What the public needs to know is that HACCP is essentially

deregulation under the guise of science. In January 1998 the USDA began transferring inspection responsibility to the industry. Federal inspectors will begin to shift to inspecting the paper produced by plans drawn up by the industry. While the plan, at the insistence of the FSIS, does include two kinds of testing—of *Salmonella* on the part of the FSIS and generic *E. coli* by the industry to establish the general level of sanitation—it was revealed shortly after the testing began that companies were coming up with uniformly negative *E. coli* tests. Their facilities appeared spotless, yet it couldn't be so. What had happened is that the USDA-authorized testing technique using sponges was actually killing the bacteria.

Consumers will also be surprised to know that finding poultry positive for *Salmonella* doesn't mean that these birds are removed from sale, but merely that they are counted toward the *Salmonella* quota. There are, in fact, numerous holes in this legislation. Shifting responsibility for safe, clean meat to industry is unlikely to either inspire confidence in consumers or produce a safe product.

It's reasonable to ask, Why is it advisable to abandon the organoleptic—the old touch, sniff, observe—inspection system at all? Why would modern consumers be any less interested in having tubercular or tapeworm-infested animals kept out of the food supply today than they were 90 years ago? On-site inspection of food animals and the slaughtering process by government inspectors protected by federal regulations from undue industry pressure is still an important part of ensuring a clean food supply, and we abandon it at our peril. Microbial testing should be added to the process, but it should not replace common sense.

Positive changes are coming at the federal level despite the powerful influence of industry and even without a single food-safety agency. The USDA is revisiting the matter of water retention in poultry (from the infamous "fecal soup" in which poultry is chilled). It is also looking steadily at the problem of contaminated eggs. It is very likely that new temperature regulations for transporting eggs will prevail, but this hardly gets at the source of the contamination problem.

Unfortunately, the HACCP approach to food safety is also likely to encourage food producers and processors to long for technological quick fixes. They can be very tempting. How easy it would be to insist that the only sure way to provide safe eggs is to supply them in a liquid pasteurized form. This makes a kind of horrible sense. Yet food is not simply fuel. It is pleasure. Eating good food is an undeniable sensual experience. Reducing it to canned, bottled, pasteurized, sterilized, and irradiated products is what David Waltner-Toews at the University of Guelph in Canada calls the "bulldozer" or "Stalinist" approach to food safety. In fact, it is tyranny. Chicken cut up in ten different ways in the supermarket isn't meaningful choice unless clean chicken is available.

Irradiation has been strongly promoted by a desperate food industry. It is routinely, and wrongly, reported that the WHO has given irradiation its unreserved blessing. In fact, there are reservations in its report, especially about lower nutrition in irradiated products. There are other serious questions. Irradiation does not, at the levels approved, destroy *Clostridium perfringens* or *Clostridium botulinum,* so irradiated products still have to be treated carefully and cooked thoroughly. Irradiation is also known to produce free radicals, which are dangerous and apparently cause cancer. Advocates of irradiation will say that cooking creates the same free radicals. But what of the cooking of irradiated products, which would multiply the effect? If the only choice is irradiation, the consumer will be paying more for a product that gives less in taste and nutrition and still has to be handled carefully and cooked thoroughly, so it is difficult to see what has been achieved. Far better to clean up the meat.

The answer is to look for the causes of contamination at the very beginning of the process rather than at the end. HACCP has an essential flaw. It looks not at critical control points where contamination could be avoided, but simply at points where it can be reduced, contained, or corrected. Thus technological responses at the end of the line are virtually mandated by an ill-conceived definition. To make way for sensible solutions to the problems of *E. coli* O157:H7, such as holding back from slaughter cattle that test positive for the microbe, or switching to hay to rid the pathogen from the cow's system, the HACCP approach needs rethinking.

It would be nice to think the goals of agribusiness were compatible with safe food, but efficiency is an inappropriate model for animal production. Animals are not machines, and it is now well established that creating stress in animals makes them more likely to harbor or to shed the pathogens that make humans sick. The role of enlightened government policy would be to restrict or limit the drive for efficiency and profit when it is counterproductive to the safety of food.

Can consumer advocacy organizations make a difference? Some groups in Washington are helping to balance the powerful presence of industry, and in the past few years they have been given a seat at the table with greater frequency. It is certainly fair to say that without their presence matters would be worse. Yet too often these groups are forced to compromise. Sometimes, standing behind the president as he announces a food-safety measure, they find themselves co-opted in an effort that may or may not be successful. They are up against powerful forces that can shape legislation apparently with ease. While supporting their efforts is a good idea, one can't simply write a check and feel secure.

As misused as science is in some contexts, it counts for a lot, when applied to public health efforts. As part of a presidential food-safety initiative, funding for surveillance and for coordination of state and national public health efforts in foodborne disease has been increased. The goal is a comprehensive electronic network, coupled with sensitive DNA laboratory testing, so that, for example, a serotype of a pathogen causing an illness in Iowa can be quickly matched to one in Kentucky. In this way a widespread outbreak from a mass-produced product might be spotted in what would otherwise seem to be sporadic and isolated cases. If epidemiology can uncover the food vehicle and the serotypes can be compared and matched, a recall can be requested, and many more individuals spared from illness. Surveillance doesn't have a sexy ring to it, and it's unlikely to stir the public's imagination enough to inspire citizen lobbying efforts, but it is essential to reducing illness and increasing accountability among food producers—which has the potential to encourage safer, cleaner food.

If change is to come, if food is to be cleaner, the impetus and energy must ultimately come from the consumer on a personal level. It must begin with a new attitude about food, a realization that eating is something more than a refueling process and that care must be exercised if what we eat is to be safe. It will involve reeducating ourselves, about foods and their origins, about seasons and their fruits, about ingredients and their uses, about shelf lives. It will require of some of us that we learn to cook and be willing to devote to the important task of feeding our families and ourselves the time it deserves. It must include a renewed assumption of responsibility, not simply to cook the contamination out of our food as we are now asked to do and must do in the short run, but to refuse to buy foods that are egregiously contaminated. And it will demand that consumers become forthright and outspoken shoppers, articulating their preferences and requirements clearly and persuasively. It can be done.

When Swedes discovered through press reports how contaminated their chickens were, they reacted at once. They stopped buying them. Consumption dropped quickly by 40 percent. Swedish chickens were then cleaned up. Today a Swedish shopper, as well as Danish shopper, can buy chickens labeled "Salmonella-free." The cleanup was due not to regulation but to the Swedish chicken industry's response to the consumer boycott of their product. By instituting rather elementary measures—clean food, clean housing, clean water, no contamination from the outside, lower stress, humane transportation, and keeping contaminated chickens out of the slaughterhouse—*Salmonella* has been eliminated and the presence of *Campylobacter,* more difficult to get rid of, has diminished considerably (13 percent contaminated as compared with 80+ percent of U.S. chickens). Clean chickens cost more, and that too will be part of the bargain. The United States has for too long had a cheap-food policy, and it is making us sick. American consumers must expect to pay more for clean food. It will be worth it. If a cheap chicken causes a case of *Campylobacter,* it can end up being very expensive indeed.

Other consumer habits that favor convenience at any cost need to be reconsidered. Asking someone else to wash and cut up vegetables you plan to eat raw is simply asking for trouble. You cannot be sure who is doing the preparation or under what conditions; this sort of trust is entirely misplaced. The small amount of time it takes to wash and cut up your own vegetables simply isn't worth the risk of leaving the tasks to others. Careful consideration should also be given to the convenience of buying prepared foods, unless you are convinced of the care and attention devoted to the process and certain that the product is very fresh.

The constant search for novelty is another factor in foodborne disease because it requires the global food trade to satisfy it. If the USDA cannot be certain that the washing facilities for lettuce on a California farm are safe—which it cannot—it is far less likely to be certain that cantaloupes washed in Mexico, grapes picked in Chile, or apples packed in South Africa are done so under sanitary conditions. No representative of the Occupational Safety and Health Administration or the USDA is on the shrimp farm in Pakistan making certain that the bathroom facilities have running water or that the harvest is packed and frozen safely.

To limit ourselves to food produced here in the United States or, more radically, to food produced within the region in which we live would mean a drastic change in the way we eat today. It would mean eating according to the seasons, as our ancestors did. That is not a bad thing. I think often about the diets of my grandparents and great-aunts and -uncles, all of whom lived to ripe old ages. Their diets were shaped precisely to the seasons. Spring began with peas and radishes and lettuces grown in cold frames with rhubarb and even wild greens. Tomatoes, corn, and beans were eaten in the summer, unless they were canned for winter consumption. Kale and leeks came in the fall. Winter squash, onions, carrots, beets, potatoes, parsnips, turnips, and cabbage all came in the summer and autumn but could be stored and eaten throughout the winter. Hog butchering, apple butter making, and cider making took place in the fall. Chickens were killed for a once-a-week treat on Sunday. This life, which I was lucky enough to share as a child, was hardly one of deprivation. We may not have known what a kiwifruit was, and strawberries had a brief season in June, but the food was fabulous. It was also fresh. And I don't recall ever getting sick.

There will be individuals who will say with conviction, "But we can't eat like that now." If we can't, the question is, "Why not? How can we say we have made any real progress if such elementary pleasures are no longer available. In fact, we *can* eat that way. People with more than postage-stamp-size gardens can plant vegetables and find out how simple it is to grow a great deal of what they eat. In rural areas local growers can be located. And cities often host farmers' markets.

What is required is some planning. And that demands that we once again think seriously about what we eat and about supplying ourselves and our families with the best and the freshest foods available. It also requires something new: the abandonment of the notion that we are somehow entitled to eat anything in the world at the precise moment the urge strikes. Even if food safety implications weren't connected to the notion, there is enormous arrogance in that attitude. There are also political implications. Encouraging underdeveloped countries to shape their agricultural practices to supply the fickle consumers in a distant marketplace rather than to meet their own needs is to destroy that country's self-reliance, an effect most shoppers buying exotic fruit seldom consider.

Consumers can begin focusing once again on local produce in season. While some might question what this has to do with food safety, it could be important. Locally grown crops travel less and are thus fresher. Fresher produce is less inviting to microbial growth, and it is certainly less likely to be contaminated with exotic microbes like *Cyclospora*. Since locally grown foods change hands less frequently, the opportunities for contamination are fewer. Most important, locally grown produce and animal products mean that a relationship of responsibility and accountability can be established between food producer and consumer. The present more common anonymous relationship between those who grow food crops and those who eat them has the opposite effect. It encourages an abstract attitude about food, an acceptance of a powerlessness on the part of consumers and detachment on the part of producers, that in itself is counterproductive to food safety. The more we consign responsibility for our food to distant suppliers, the less control we ultimately have over what we eat.

The present alternatives are limited and unpalatable. The choices we are being offered are either to accept that food in the future will be pasteurized, sterilized, and irradiated or to turn our kitchens into biohazard labs. The first is unappealing, and the second is impossible to achieve successfully. Accidents happen frequently in the actual biohazard labs handling these microbes, and American kitchens cannot be expected to maintain laboratory conditions. Real life happens in our kitchens. Children play, animals run in and out, and a confused and hectic atmosphere often prevails in busy households; food preparation may be undertaken by young people who haven't the training and can't be expected to assume the stringent adult responsibilities that safe food handling now seems to demand. To make the consumer responsible for safely cooking the contamination out of foods while dodging cross-contamination is asking too much.

The third, unspoken choice is to create change. There is no reason why the Swedish Chicken Revolution could not take place in the United States. Several factors are preventing it. All can be surmounted.

First, consumers must understand just how contaminated certain foods have become and decide that the present level of contamination of many raw animal products is unacceptable.

Then they must appreciate that, contrary to what the industry says, these products do not have to be so thoroughly contaminated. Contamination can be reduced, sometimes in simple ways. The Swedish approach is to make certain that no contaminated poultry reaches the processing environment; the U.S. approach is to focus on reducing contamination by means such as increasing the chlorine in the infamous poultry "fecal soup" chilling water. There are methods that work to reduce contamination at the source. New studies show that merely feeding cattle hay for five days before slaughter could eliminate the dangerous pathogen *E. coli* O157:H7. American beef producers should be given every encouragement and incentive to implement this practice. The Dutch and British governments are embarking on a course of reducing or eliminating the *Salmonella* in eggs, and their approach could be implemented here as well.

Key to achieving cleaner food is allowing and encouraging food producers to use food safety as a marketing strategy. While the USDA has no authority to demand that feedlots switch cattle to the safer hay diet before slaughter, a beef-processing plant could advertise on its hamburger that its cattle had been switched to reduce *E. coli* contamination. Savvy consumers could then select that beef over one without that assurance. Eggs could be labeled "From salmonella-free hens," or chickens labeled "Salmonella-free" or "Campylobacter-reduced."

In the very best supermarkets across America, fruits and vegetables often come with signs indicating their origin. Occasionally it is even possible in the most responsible food markets to learn precisely from which farm the produce came. This is the way to shop, and consumers must lobby to make certain that labeling is not discouraged or even forbidden by regulation. Demanding consumers are responsible for the availability of labeling in the few stores that provide it. When it isn't available, consumers should ask supermarket clerks and produce managers to make the information available. Even in states where particular labeling is required by law, large supermarket chains routinely flout the requirement. With pinched state budgets, enforcement is ultimately up to the consumer. With clear and accurate labeling, good producers will be rewarded for providing good products.

Consumers hold the ultimate weapon in this battle. We still can choose where our money will be spent and, indeed, whether it will be spent. Our demands can shape our food world. But consumers have to care. We have to be knowledgeable. We have to be willing to pay more for good foods.

While high prices are no inherent guarantee of safe food, extremely low cost can be a warning sign of contaminated food. Pressures in the poultry industry to produce chickens for the lowest possible price with the highest profit margin have led to practices that increase the risk of contamination. The same is true for hamburger and for many other foods. Producers can still be efficient while employing tactics that reduce contamination, but they may have to charge more, and thus they need to be able to tout the measures they take to provide this margin of safety. Consumers need to be educated enough to know what measures are important and be willing to pay for them. A certain amount of faith can then be invested in the operation of the marketplace, but only when a free-flow of information will enable consumers to make intelligent choices. At the moment, however, the policies of the USDA seem designed to put obstacles in the way of consumers' gaining this information—at least in discouraging point-of-origin labeling and the use of food safety as a marketing strategy. The food industry itself also discourages its members from using food safety as a marketing strategy, presumably because those who don't participate will look bad.

Consumer pressure can change this. Why not stop buying hamburger until it's clear precisely where it comes from, whether it was purchased by the retailer already coarse ground, precisely how old it is, what kind of meat it contains, whether it contains that mystery substance, imported ground beef, and whether efforts to eliminate pathogenic organisms were incorporated in its production?

The point is to think anew about food and food safety and to apply a basic understanding of microbes and their habits to purchasing food, preparing it, and consuming it. Respect for our bodies and what we put into them goes without saying. One thing is increasingly certain. Food can no longer be approached with the trusting assumption that someone else has done the worrying for us. If we want clean food, we are going to have to work for it.

Appendix: Sources

The World Wide Web is a good resource for those who want even more specific information on food safety. Some of the sources are good, some not so good. Use your judgment and common sense. University sources are not always as reliable as one might expect from the perspective of the most up-to-date information. The government sources listed here are usually right on top of the changing nature of foodborne disease. Industry sources naturally put things in the best light possible.

Basic Government Sources of Information

The **Centers for Disease Control and Prevention (CDC)** is an agency of the Department of Health and Human Services headquartered in Atlanta, Georgia. Its aim is the promotion of health and quality of life by preventing and controlling disease, injury, and disability. To this end it tracks and investigates the causes of human disease and is the ultimate source for the latest information. Its publication, the *Morbidity and Mortality Weekly Report (MMWR)*, which surely wins the contest for most unappealing name ever created, is nevertheless a vital document for those who keep up with the changing nature of human disease. The Centers' web site is a treasure of information on human disease, and the information on specific diseases or for travelers is reliable and up-to-date.

Centers for Disease Control and Prevention
1600 Clifton Road MS D-25
Atlanta, GA 30333
Tel: 404-639-3311

Public inquiries: 1-800-311-3435
Web sites
General: cdc.gov
Public information: cdc.gov/od/oc/media

The **United States Department of Agriculture (USDA)** is a huge agency whose mission is to "Enhance the quality of life for the American people by supporting production of agriculture." This gives it a built-in conflict of interest when it comes to ensuring that those products are safe, a problem it attempts to overcome through a separate division for food safety called the Food Safety and Inspection Service (FSIS). Nevertheless, the conflict automatically calls into question some of its decisions and its reporting of foodborne disease.

Responsibility for food safety is confusingly divided among several federal agencies. The USDA is responsible for the safety of raw animal products, such as poultry, pork, beef, and eggs, although it shares some of the responsibility for eggs with the FDA.

The information for consumers on how they can keep themselves safe is accurate, instructive, and very detailed. There are six pages, for instance, on what kind of food thermometer to buy and how to use one safely. The Web is the best—and virtually the only way—to access this information, which can be printed out. Many libraries now have web access if you don't own a computer yourself. There is also a Meat and Poultry Hotline.

Food Safety and Inspection Service
United States Department of Agriculture
Washington, DC 20250-3700
USDA/FSIS Meat and Poultry Hotline: 1-800-535-4555
FSIS Food Safety Education and Communications Staff,
Public Outreach and Communication: Tel: 202-720-9352;
Fax: 202-720-9063
Web sites
General: usda.gov
FSIS: fsis.usda.gov
Consumer food-safety publications: fsis.usda.gov/OA/pubs/con sumerpubs.htm

The **Food and Drug Administration (FDA),** in its own words, "touches the lives of virtually every American every day. For it is FDA's job to see that the food we eat is safe and wholesome, the cosmetics we use won't hurt us, the medicines and medical devices we use are safe and effective, and that radiation-emitting products such as microwave ovens won't do us harm. Feed and drugs for pets and farm animals also come under FDA scrutiny. FDA also ensures that all of these products are labeled truthfully with the information that people need to use them properly." Actually, the food the FDA is responsible for, through its Center for Food Safety and Applied Nutrition (CFSAN), does not include raw animal products, except for milk and seafood. Its description on its web site of how well it carries out the inspection of foods is overly optimistic. (As little as 2 percent of imported foods are spot-checked, and then only if there have been problems with those foods.) However, the material on food safety and food pathogens provided on the FDA web site is generally excellent. Their *Bad Bug Book* is a wonderful source for information on foodborne pathogens, although it needs updating.

FDA (HFE-88)
5600 Fishers Lane
Rockville, MD 20857
Tel: 1-800-532-4440

Center for Food Safety and Applied Nutrition
200 C Street, SW
Washington, DC 20204

CFSAN Food Information and Seafood Hotline: 1-800-FDA-4010
Emergency number for use in a case of foodborne illness or a drug product that has been tampered with, staffed 24 hours a day: 301-443-1240.
Web site: www.fda.gov

The National Food Safety Initiative is a joint effort of these federal agencies and the Environmental Protection Agency. Their web site is a clearinghouse for a wide variety of information on food safety.

Web site: vm.cfsan.fda.gov~dms/fs-toc.html

Government and Public Partnership

Fight Bac® is a joint endeavor of the federal government agencies that deal with food safety and the food industry. This is a program to get information to the public on how to handle contaminated foods safely, with the goal of reducing foodborne disease. All the information is copyrighted, but brochures, posters, and other attractively produced material can be purchased for distribution by organizations, businesses, and individuals. The information is accurate but presented with a slight industry slant. The same information, minus the slant, is available without the copyright on the FSIS web site. However, the Fight Bac® web site has excellent links to the sites of its industry members, and some information on these sites cannot be found elsewhere.

Web site: fightbac.org/
Materials can be ordered via the web or from
Partnership for Food Safety Education
800 Connecticut Avenue, NW
Washington, DC 20006
Tel: 202-429-4550

Nonprofit Organizations

These organizations generally support consumer interests and advocate in their behalf in the public arena, but each has a specific focus.

Safe Tables Our Priority (S.T.O.P.) was organized by families and friends of some of the first *E. coli* victims but has now extended its reach to all foodborne pathogens. In its own words, "S.T.O.P. is a nonprofit organization composed of victims of foodborne illness, their families and friends and concerned individuals and organizations who recognize the threat of emerging microorganisms in our food supply. We share a strong belief that most foodborne injuries and deaths are preventable in the United States today. By taking action, we want our experiences to be catalysts for positive change. S.T.O.P. is unique among consumer organizations in its composition of and support for victims. If you believe you are suffering from a foodborne illness or if you think you have had one, contact S.T.O.P."

E-mail: feedback@stop-usa.org
Web site: http://www.stop-usa.org/

The **Center for Science in the Public Interest (CSPI)** was founded in Washington, D.C., in 1971 by three Ph.D. scientists who had met a year earlier while all were working at Ralph Nader's Center for the Study of Responsive Law. They envisioned a consumer advocacy organization based on science. Today they tackle many food issues and publish the *Nutrition Action Healthletter*, which both informs and coordinates consumer action. They also have an excellent web site that focuses specifically on the repressive laws that allow food suppliers to sue those who criticize their food products.

Center for Science in the Public Interest
1875 Connecticut Avenue, NW, #300
Washington, DC 20009
Tel: 202-332-9110; Fax: 202-265-4954
Web site: cspinet.org

Nutrition Action Healthletter subscriptions:
Nutrition Action Circulation Department
1875 Connecticut Avenue, NW, #300
Washington, DC 20009-5728

Public Citizen is the organization founded by Ralph Nader in 1971 to be, as it says, "the consumer's eyes and ears in Washington. With the support of more than 150,000 people like you, we fight for safer drugs and medical devices, cleaner and safer energy sources, a cleaner environment, fair trade, and a more open and democratic government."

According to their web site, "We stand up for you against thousands of special interest lobbyists in Washington—well-heeled agents for drug companies, the automakers, big energy interests, and the like. Our budget is small by comparison. But Public Citizen is respected and effective, precisely because we accept no government or corporate support. We speak only for you." It focuses on the impact of trade on food safety.

Public Citizen
1600 20th Street, NW
Washington, DC 20009
Tel: 202-833-3000; Fax: 202-296-1727
To join: 1-800-289-3787

Mothers & Others is a national nonprofit education organization that "works to promote consumer choices which are safe and ecologically sustainable for this generation and the next. By providing strategies that can reduce individual and community consumption of natural resources and by mobilizing consumers to seek sustainable choices, we aim to effect lasting protection of public health and the environment." The group puts out an excellent newsletter, *The Green Guide*, which often covers food issues.

Mothers & Others for a Livable Planet
40 West 20th Street
New York, NY 10011-4211
Web site: igc.org/mothers

Campaign for Food Safety (formerly known as the Pure Food Campaign) is a grassroots organization run by Ronnie Cummins that coordinates and inspires consumer activism in the fight for clean food.

Campaign for Food Safety
860 Highway 61
Little Marais, Minnesota 55614
Activist or media inquiries: Tel: 218-226-4164; Fax: 218-226-4157

Those with E-mail can subscribe free to his E-mail newsletter by sending an E-mail to majordomo@mr.net with the message, "subscribe pure-food-action."

Food and Water is one of the strongest advocacy groups, so intense, independent, and committed in its efforts that it makes some of the other organizations wary. No punches are pulled at Food and Water, and it doesn't flinch from going after icons if necessary. But the information in its handsome and eloquently written journal is great, and its efforts get results. Consumer activism is its raison d'être. The director is a neo-Luddite, and it doesn't have a web site.

Food and Water
389 Vermont Route 215
Walden, Vermont 05873

Sources for Oral Rehydration Salt Packets Prepared to WHO Standards

Travel Medicine, Inc is both a fascinating catalogue as well as a source for smaller quantities of oral rehydration packets. They can be reached by mail at:

351 Pleasant Street, Suite 312
Northampton, MA 01060
413-584-0381
E-mail: travmed@travmed.com
Tel: 800-872-8633 (800-TRAV-MED)
Web site: http://www.travmed.com

These companies prefer to sell in bulk, although Jianas has a travel box of 20 packets. A parents organization or group could purchase a case and divide it among themselves, or ask your pharmacy to order from these companies.

Cera Products, Inc.
8265-I Patuxent Range Road
Jessup, MD 20794
Tel: 1-888-237-2598; 301-490-4941
Fax: 301-490-4942

Jianas Brothers
2533 Southwest Boulevard
Kansas City, MO 64108
Tel: 816-421-2880; Fax: 816-421-2883

Other Sources: Camping supply stores as well as catalogs for serious camping often supply first aid kits containing ORS packets or provide the packets themselves in smaller quantities.

Bibliography

The science and ecology of foodborne disease were examined in my book, *Spoiled* (BasicBooks, 1997; Penguin, 1998). *It Was Probably Something You Ate* is intended as a follow-up, with the specific goal of being an easy-to-access and useful reference for the consumer. Some readers, however, may want to pursue some aspect of the subject in more technical detail, and for them I am including a list of some of the publications that I used to research this book. For information on incubation times for particular pathogens, the FDA and the CDC web sites were particularly helpful and are listed in the resource section.

GENERAL

The following acronyms are used in this bibliography:

AJPH—*American Journal of Public Health*
JAMA—*Journal of the American Medical Association*
JAVMA—*Journal of the American Veterinary Medical Association*
MMWR—*Morbidity and Mortality Weekly Report*

Centers for Disease Control and Prevention, *Conference on Emerging Foodborne Disease, Emerging Infectious Diseases*, 1997; 3(4):415–584.
Centers for Disease Control and Prevention, *Reports of the 44tth, 45th, 46th, and 47th Epidemic Intelligence Service Conference*, 1995, 1996, 1997, 1998.
Conference Proceedings, Tracking Foodborne Pathogens from Farm to Table: Data Needs to Evaluate Control Options. United States Department of Agriculture, January 9–10, 1995.

Lederberg, Joshua, Robert E. Shope, and Stanley C. Oaks, Jr., editors, *Emerging Infections: Microbial Threats to Health in the United States.* Institute of Medicine, National Academy Press, 1992.

National Research Council, *Ensuring Safe Food: From Production to Consumption.* Institute of Medicine, National Academy Press, 1998.

Rampton, Sheldon, and John Stauber, *Mad Cow U.S.A.: Could the Nightmare Happen Here?* Monroe, Maine: Common Courage Press, 1997.

Rhodes, Richard, *Deadly Feasts: Tracking the Secrets of a Terrifying New Plague.* Simon & Schuster, 1997.

Roizman, Bernard, editor, *Infectious Diseases in an Age of Change: The Impact of Human Ecology and Behavior on Disease Transmission.* National Academy of Sciences, National Academy Press, 1995.

Task Force Report, Foodborne Pathogens: Risks and Consequences. Council for Agricultural Science and Technology (CAST), September 1994.

Todd, Ewen, Foodborne Illness: Epidemiology of Foodborne Illness: North America. *Lancet* (UK), 1990; 336:788–790.

CAMPYLOBACTER

Allos, Ban Mishu, and Martin J. Blaser, Campylobacter jejuni and the Expanding Spectrum of Related Infections. *Clinical Infectious Diseases*, 1995; 20:1092–1101.

Blaser, Martin J., Elizabeth Sazie, and L. Paul Williams, Jr., The Influence of Immunity on Raw Milk–Associated Campylobacter Infection. *JAMA*, 1987; 257:43–46.

Deming, Michael S., Robert V. Tauxe, Paul A. Blake et al., Campylobacter enteritis at a University: Transmission from Eating Chicken and from Cats. *American Journal of Epidemiology*, 1987; 126:526–534.

Istre, Gregory R., Martin J. Blaser, Pamela Shillam, and Richard S. Hopkins, Campylobacter enteritis Associated with Undercooked Barbecued Chicken. *AJPH*, 1984; 74:1265–1267.

Kotula, Kathryn L., and Yoga Pandya, Bacterial Contamination of Broiler Chickens before Scalding. *Journal of Food Protection*, 1995; 58:1326–1329.

Mead, G. C., Problems of Producing Safe Poultry: Discussion Paper. *Journal of the Royal Society of Medicine* (UK), 1993; 86:39–42.

The National Advisory Committee on Microbiological Criteria for Foods, Campylobacter jejuni/coli. *Journal of Food Protection*, 1994; 57:1101–1121.

Smith, James L., Arthritis, Guillain-Barré Syndrome, and Other Sequelae of Campylobacter jejuni enteritis. *Journal of Food Protection*, 1995; 58:1153–1170.

Wood, Rachael C., Kirstine L. MacDonald, and Michael T. Osterholm, Campylobacter enteritis Outbreaks Associated with Drinking Raw Milk During Youth Activities. *JAMA*, 1992; 268:3328–3330.

SALMONELLA

Allos, Ban Mishu, Jane Koehler, Lisa A. Lee et al., Outbreaks of Salmonella enteritidis Infections in the United States, 1985–1991. *Journal of Infectious Diseases*, 1994; 169:547–552.

Bryan, Frank L., and Michael P. Doyle, Health Risks and Consequences of Salmonella and Campylobacter jejuni in Raw Poultry. *Journal of Food Protection*, 1995; 58:326–344.

Centers for Disease Control and Prevention, Outbreak of Salmonella enteritidis Infection Associated with Consumption of Raw Shell Eggs. *MMWR* leads in *JAMA*, 1992; 267:3263–3264.

Hennessy, Thomas W., Craig W. Hedberg, Laurence Slutsker et al., A National Outbreak of Salmonella enteritidis Infections from Ice Cream. *New England Journal of Medicine*, 1996; 334:1281–1286.

Humphrey, T. J., M. Greenwood, R. J. Gilbert, B. Rowe, and P. A. Chapman, The Survival of Salmonellas in Shell Eggs Cooked Under Simulated Domestic Conditions. *Epidemiology of Infection*, 1989; 103:35–45.

James, William O., W. Oliver Williams, Jr., John C. Prucha, Ralph Johnston, and Walter Christensen, Profile of Selected Bacterial Counts and Salmonella Prevalence on Raw Poultry in a Poultry Slaughter Establishment. *JAVMA*, 1992;200:57–59.

Rodrigue, C. C., R. V. Tauxe, and B. Rowe, International Increase in Salmonella enteritidis: A New Pandemic? *Epidemiology of Infection*, 1990; 105:21–27.

Ryan, Caroline A., Mary K Nickels, Nancy T. Hargrett-Bean et al., Massive Outbreak of Antimicrobial-Resistant Salmonellosis Traced to Pasteurized Milk. *JAMA*, 1987:3269–3274.

St. Louis, Michael E., Dale L. Morse, Morris E. Potter et al., The Emergence of Grade A Eggs as a Major Source of Salmonella enteritidis Infections. *JAMA*, 1988; 259:2103–2107.

SALMONELLA DT104

Glynn, M. Kathleen, Cheryl Bopp, Wallis Dewitt et al., Emergence of Multidrug-Resistant Salmonella enterica Serotype typhimurium DT104 Infections in the United States. *New England Journal of Medicine*, 1998; 338(19):1333–1338.

ESCHERICHIA COLI O157:H7

Ackers, Marta-Louise, Barbara E. Mahon, Ellen Leahy et al., An Out-
break of Escherichia coli O157:H6 Infections Associated with Leaf
Lettuce Consumption. *The Journal of Infectious Diseases*, 1998;
177:1588–1593.
Diez-Gonzalez, Francisco, Todd R. Callaway, Menas G. Kizoulis, and
James B. Russell, Grain Feeding and the Dissemination of Acid-
Resistant Escherichia coli from Cattle. *Science*, 1998: September 11;
281: 1666–1668.
Armstrong, Gregory L., Jill Hollingsworth, and J. Glenn Morris, Jr.,
Emerging Foodborne Pathogens: Escherichia coli O157:H7 as a
Model of Entry of a New Pathogen into the Food Supply of the
Developed World. *Epidemiologic Reviews*, 1995;18:1–15.
Griffin, Patricia M., *Escherichia coli O157:H7 and other Enterohemorrhagic
Escherichia coli*. Chapter 52, Infections of the Gastrointestinal Tract.
Raven Press, 1995.
Karmali, M. A., and A. G. Goglio, editors, *Recent Advances in Verocytotoxin
Producing Escherichia coli Infections*. Elsevier, 1994.

SHIGELLA

Centers for Disease Control and Prevention, Outbreak of Shigella
flexneri 2a Infections on a Cruise Ship. *MMWR*, 1994; 43(35).
Centers for Disease Control and Prevention, Shigella sonnei Outbreak
Associated with Contaminated Drinking Water—Island Park, Idaho,
August 1995. *MMWR*, 1996; 45(11):229–231.

CYCLOSPORA

Centers for Disease Control and Prevention, Outbreaks of Cyclospora
cayetanensis Infection—United States, 1996. *MMWR*, 1996; 45(25).
Huang, P., J. T. Wever, D. M. Sosin et al., The First Reported Outbreak
of Diarrheal Illness Associated with Cyclospora in the United States.
Annals of Internal Medicine, 1995; 123:409–414.
Ortega, Y. R., C. R. Sterling, R. H. Gilman, V. A. Cama, and F. Diaz, Cy-
clospora Species—a New Protozoan Pathogen of Humans. *New
England Journal of Medicine*, 1993; 328:1308–1312.

CLOSTRIDIUM BOTULINUM

Centers for Disease Control and Prevention, Foodborne Botulism—Oklahoma, 1994. *MMWR*, 1995; 44.

Macdonald, Kristine L., Robert F. Spengler, Charles L. Hatheway et al., Type A Botulism from Sautéed Onions: Clinical and Epidemiologic Observations. *JAMA*, 1985; 253:1275–1278.

St. Louis, Michael E., *Botulism.* In A. S. Evans and P. Brachman, editors, *Bacterial Infections of Humans: Epidemiology and Control.* Plenum Publishing, 2nd ed., 1991; 115–131.

St. Louis, Michael E., Shaun H. S. Peck, David Bowering et al., Botulism from Chopped Garlic: Delayed Recognition of a Major Outbreak. *Annals of Internal Medicine*, 1988; 108:363–368.

Seals, Jerry E., John D. Snyder, Timm A. Edell, Charles L. Hatheway, Carl J. Johnson, Richard C. Swanson, and James M. Hughes, Restaurant-Associated Type A Botulism: Transmission by Potato Salad. *American Journal of Epidemiology*, 1981; 113:436–444.

Shaffer, Nathan, Robert B. Wainwright, John P. Middaugh, and Robert V. Tauxe, Botulism Among Alaska Natives: The Role of Changing Food Preparation and Consumption Practices. *The Western Journal of Medicine*, 1990; 153:390–393.

HEPATITIS A

Centers for Disease Control and Prevention, Hepatitis A Associated with Consumption of Frozen Strawberries—Michigan, March 1997. *MMWR*, 1997; 46: 288, 295.

CIGUATERA

Centers for Disease Control and Prevention, Ciguatera Fish Poisoning, 1997. *MMWR*, 1998; 47(33).

Centers for Disease Control and Prevention, Ciguatera Fish Poisoning—Florida, 1991. *MMWR*, 1993; 42(21).

VIBRIO VULNIFICUS

Centers for Disease Control and Prevention, Vibrio vulnificus Infections Associated with Eating Raw Oysters—Los Angeles, 1996. *MMWR*, 1995; 44(29).

Centers for Disease Control and Prevention, Vibrio vulnificus Infections Associated with Raw Oyster Consumption. *MMWR*, 1993; 42(21).

VIBRIO CHOLERA

Motes, Miles, Angelo DePaola, Sabrina Zywno van Ginkel, and Merrill McPhearson, Occurrence of Toxigenic Vibrio Cholerae O1 in Oysters in Mobile Bay, Alabama: An Ecological Investigation. 1994; 57:975–980.

CRYPTOSPORIDIUM

MacKenzie, William R., Neil J. Hoxie, Mary E. Proctor et al., A Massive Outbreak in Milwaukee of Cryptosporidium Infection Transmitted Through the Public Water Supply. *New England Journal of Medicine*, 1994; 331:161–167.

BOVINE SPONGIFORM ENCEPHALOPATHY

Collinge, J., C. L. Sidle, J. Meads, J. Ironside, and A. F. Hill, Molecular Analysis of Prion Strain Variation and the Etiology of "New Variant" CJD. *Nature*, 1996; 383: 685–690.

Wilesmith, John W., Gerald A. H. Wells, M. P. Cranwell, and J. B. M. Ryan, Bovine Spongiform Encephalopathy: Epidemological Studies. *Veterinary Record*, December 17, 1988; 638–644.

Will, R. G., J. W. Ironside, M. Zeidler et al., A New Variant of Creutzfeldt-Jakob Disease in the United Kingdom. *Lancet* (UK), 1996; 347:921–925.

PRODUCE

Beuchat, Larry R., Pathogenic Microorganisms Associated with Fresh Produce. *Journal of Food Protection*, 1996; 59:204–216.

Index

FOR THE BEST IN PAPERBACKS, LOOK FOR THE

In every corner of the world, on every subject under the sun, Penguin represents quality and variety—the very best in publishing today.

For complete information about books available from Penguin—including Puffins, Penguin Classics, and Arkana—and how to order them, write to us at the appropriate address below. Please note that for copyright reasons the selection of books varies from country to country.

In the United Kingdom: Please write to *Dept. EP, Penguin Books Ltd, Bath Road, Harmondsworth, West Drayton, Middlesex UB7 0DA.*

In the United States: Please write to *Penguin Putnam Inc., P.O. Box 12289 Dept. B, Newark, New Jersey 07101-5289* or call 1-800-788-6262.

In Canada: Please write to *Penguin Books Canada Ltd, 10 Alcorn Avenue, Suite 300, Toronto, Ontario M4V 3B2.*

In Australia: Please write to *Penguin Books Australia Ltd, P.O. Box 257, Ringwood, Victoria 3134.*

In New Zealand: Please write to *Penguin Books (NZ) Ltd, Private Bag 102902, North Shore Mail Centre, Auckland 10.*

In India: Please write to *Penguin Books India Pvt Ltd, 11 Panchsheel Shopping Centre, Panchsheel Park, New Delhi 110 017.*

In the Netherlands: Please write to *Penguin Books Netherlands bv, Postbus 3507, NL-1001 AH Amsterdam.*

In Germany: Please write to *Penguin Books Deutschland GmbH, Metzlerstrasse 26, 60594 Frankfurt am Main.*

In Spain: Please write to *Penguin Books S. A., Bravo Murillo 19, 1° B, 28015 Madrid.*

In Italy: Please write to *Penguin Italia s.r.l., Via Benedetto Croce 2, 20094 Corsico, Milano.*

In France: Please write to *Penguin France, Le Carré Wilson, 62 rue Benjamin Baillaud, 31500 Toulouse.*

In Japan: Please write to *Penguin Books Japan Ltd, Kaneko Building, 2-3-25 Koraku, Bunkyo-Ku, Tokyo 112.*

In South Africa: Please write to *Penguin Books South Africa (Pty) Ltd, Private Bag X14, Parkview, 2122 Johannesburg.*